Functional Disorders and
Medically Unexplained Symptoms

Functional Disorders and Medically Unexplained Symptoms

Assessment and treatment

Edited by
Per Fink and Marianne Rosendal

The Research Clinic for Functional
Disorders and Psychosomatics
Aarhus University Hospital
2015

Functional Disorders and Medically Unexplained Symptoms
Edited by Per Fink and Marianne Rosendal
English translation by Morten Pilegaard
© The authors and Aarhus University Press
Layout and typesetting: Narayana Press
Cover design: Sparre Grafisk
Printed at Narayana Press
Printed in Denmark 2015

ISBN 978-87-7124-851-7

Aarhus University Press
www.unipress.dk

In collaboration with

The Research Clinic for Functional Disorders and Psychosomatics
Aarhus University Hospital
DK-8000 Aarhus C
Denmark

International distribution
UK & Eire:
Gazelle Book Services Ltd.
White Cross Mills
Hightown, Lancaster, LA1 4XS
United Kingdom
www.gazellebookservices.co.uk

North America:
ISD
70 Enterprise Drive, Suite 2
Bristol, CT 06010
USA
www.isdistribution.com

Published with the financial support of
Aarhus University Research Foundation

Table of content

Editors

Per Fink

PhD from Aarhus University in 1993 with a thesis about the relationship between the prevalence of mental and physical diseases, and in 1997 Doctor of Medicine with a dissertation on chronic somatisation. Since 1999 employed as a senior doctor at The Research Clinic for Functional Disorders, Aarhus University Hospital, and the same year employed as a Clinical Associate Professor at the University of Aarhus. In 2009 Per Fink was appointed professor.

Per Fink has published around 130 scientific articles in international journals, textbook chapters in Denmark and abroad, and has lectured extensively at home and abroad. Per Fink's research is devoted to the study of functional diseases, and together with Marianne Rosendal and Tomas Toft, he has devised an educational programme for general practitioners and other doctors in the treatment of functional disorders, the so-called TERM model.

Per Fink is also a co-founder of the European Organization for Liaison Psychiatry and Psychosomatics, and is a Fellow of the Academy of Psychosomatic Medicine in the United States. He helped create the Interest Group on Liaison Psychiatry of the Danish Society of Psychiatry and was the Group's first President. Per Fink has won several research prizes, among others he was awarded The Alan Stoudemire Award for Innovation and Excellence in Psychosomatic Medicine Education in 2007 for his work with the TERM model.

Marianne Rosendal

MSc from Odense University in 1989 and a general practice specialist in 1996. After some years in general practice, Marianne Rosendal acquired a PhD degree at the Faculty of Health Sciences, Aarhus University in 2003. Her research focused on the treatment of medically unexplained symptoms and functional disorders in general practice. From 2003 to 2006, Marianne Rosendal served as a general practitioner in her own practice, but since 2006 she has been a senior researcher at The Research Unit for General Practice, Aarhus University, where she has also participated in quality development in relation to general practice.

Together with Per Fink and Tomas Toft, Marianne Rosendal helped lay the foundation for the treatment programme, the TERM model, and has ever since participated in its further development and dissemination. Marianne Rosendal has also been involved in the development of classification systems in relation to symptoms and functional disorders in general practice. In that connection, she has served on the working groups under the WHO and Wonca (the World Organization of Practitioners). As part of her research and teaching of functional disorders, Marianne Rosendal coordinated the work to develop a clinical guide on this topic which was published by the Danish College of General Practitioners in 2013.

Authors

Andreas Schröder, PhD, MD

Senior registrar, senior researcher
The Research Clinic for Functional Disorders,
Aarhus University Hospital, Denmark

Ann Ostenfeld-Rosenthal, PhD, MA

Associate professor
Department of Public Health
University of Southern Denmark

Charlotte Ulrikka Rask, PhD, MD

Clinical associate professor, postdoctoral fellow
The Research Clinic for Functional Disorders,
Aarhus University Hospital, Denmark

Lene Toscano, MD

Specialist in General Medicine
The Research Clinic for Functional Disorders,
Aarhus University Hospital, Denmark

Marianne Rosendal, PhD, MD

Senior researcher
The Research Unit for General Practice
Aarhus University, Denmark

Mette Bech Risør, PhD, MA

Researcher
The Research Unit for General Practice, Department of Social Medicine
University of Tromso, Norway

Per Fink, PhD, MD, DmSc

Director
The Research Clinic for Functional Disorders,
Aarhus University Hospital, Denmark

Tomas Toft, PhD, MD

Consultant
The Psychiatric Ward
Odense University Hospital, Denmark

Trine Dalsgaard, PhD, MA

Anthropologist, Denmark

Preface

Physical symptoms are common, but some people experience a condition of actual *bodily distress*, where the symptoms themselves cause an illness, although the symptoms do not fit into any known psychiatric or somatic disease pattern. Besides being a symptom of a possible physical disease, somatic symptoms may, in some cases, be an expression of physical, mental or social stress or strain.

Specific treatment is rarely necessary, but in some cases the symptoms become debilitating. We have previously found it difficult to treat some of the individuals with these symptoms, and doctors may have felt powerless. For this reason, some patients with bodily distress were perceived as difficult. As a doctor, you want to give these patients the same quality of treatment as that which is offered to other patients. The purpose of this initiative is to improve the doctors' ability to recognise and prevent inappropriate illness behaviour, both on the doctors' own part and among patients, and to improve our treatment of this patient group

The training programme has been prepared by the Research Clinic for Functional Disorders, Aarhus University Hospital, in collaboration with the Research Unit for General Practice, Aarhus University. In addition to this manual, the programme consists of an intensive course in which the various elements of the treatment model are trained by means of practical exercises. Separate training materials have been designed for participants and teachers. The training programme was originally developed for general practitioners[1] (GPs), but the current version has been modified to further its use by all

---

1   Corresponds to family physician

non-psychiatric doctors. The training programme focuses on diagnosing and treatment of functional disorders, but many of the techniques taught are of a general nature and can therefore be of much benefit in the treatment of other mental disorders as well as in general everyday clinical practice. The programme was originally developed in connection with the FIP study[2] (prevention of functional disorders and inappropriate illness behaviour in general practice), which was an interdisciplinary collaboration involving The Research Clinic for Functional Disorders, Aarhus University Hospital, The Research Unit for General Practice, Aarhus University, The Department of Ethnography and Social Anthropology, Aarhus University, and The Department of Psychology, University of Aarhus. This project has worked closely with the study "Somatising patients in general practice"[3] which emanated from the Quality Improvement Committee Q2, Vejle County, and the Research Unit and Department for General Practice, Aarhus University. Our appreciation goes to the general practitioners Frede Olesen, Hans Kallerup, Laurits Ovesen, Jette Schjødt, Sven Ingerslev, Mogens Tuborgh, Annette Vibæk Lund, Martin Holm, Kaj Sparle Christensen, Jette Møller Nielsen and Lene Agersnap, and psychiatrist Lene Søndergaard Nielsen, MSc in Psychology Lisbeth Frostholm for reading, commenting and actively participating in the development of this programme. We also wish to thank Professor Linda Gask, University of Manchester, who inspired the design of the original course programme. Furthermore, we wish to thank the many doctors who have completed the course and provided valuable feedback and ideas for improvement.

Some parts of the training programme build on *The Reattribution Model* developed in Manchester by Professor David Goldberg and Associate Professor Linda Gask in the early 1980s [1-11]. However, we have significantly modified the original model and added several new elements. The name has

2   The FIP study was funded by: The National Research Council's multidisciplinary research programme on health promotion and prevention research, which was part of a cross-Council programme for health research (grant No. 9801278) and the Quality Development Committee for General Practice in Aarhus County.

3   The project was funded by the Quality Development Committee for General Practice, Q2, The Vejle County Medical Scientific Research Fund, the Fund for funding of research in general practice and health care, and the General Practitioners' Training and Development Fund and Sara Kirstine Dalby Krabbe's Scholarship.

therefore been changed to the TERM Model (*The Extended Reattribution and Management Model*).

The most significant changes are:
a) General interview technique has been incorporated into the model.
b) A clearer discrimination is made between the different principles. For example, we emphasise only to use active listening and assessment in the first phase. Many doctors tend to be over "efficient", to give advice and to offer explanations too quickly, which is very inappropriate when dealing with somatising patients.
c) Questions about mental illness, functional level and expectations to treatment, etc. are added as independent items.
d) The biological basis of somatoform disorders is central to the explanatory model.
e) We have added a guide for follow-up treatment.
f) We have added a guide for treatment or management of sub-acute and chronic somatising patients.
g) The project and the educational programme are described in detail for documentation purposes.

Some parts of the current version have been thoroughly revised compared to the first edition. The book and the treatment model have been rewritten to target all doctors. Chapters 1-9 on the theoretical background have been reviewed and updated with the latest knowledge. We have added a new Part III, which describes the follow-up care, and a Part IV on children and adolescents. Moreover, we have included anonymous patient stories and cases based on the authors' experiences. All the patients' identities have been blurred to a degree that they will not be recognisable by either themselves or by people who know them. The patient stories remain representative of the issues exemplified and illustrated.

The overall goals of this training programme are
1. To give doctors a better understanding of the characteristics of functional disorders.
2. To improve doctors' capability to diagnose functional disorders.
3. To improve doctors' capability of:

- terminating ineffective treatment or facilitating further treatment
- treating functional symptoms and less severe cases of functional disorders
- managing chronic cases of functional disorders.

Reading guide

Part I (Chapters 1-8) provides a theoretical introduction to the subject of functional disorders. This knowledge lies at the root of any treatment of patients. Part II (Chapters 9-11) describes the treatment based on the TERM Model. Part III (Chapters 12-13) describes the follow-up treatment. Part IV (Chapter 15) describes the particularities of children and adolescents. Part V contains Chapters 16-17 which is supplementary reading about the cultural and historical background. At the back of the book there is an appendix, which contains forms for evaluation and treatment; also, a list of supplementary materials, including a website and an index.

Abbreviations used

BDS	Bodily Distress Syndrome (a novel unifying diagnostic category)
BDS, single-organ type	BDS type characterised by symptoms primarily from one bodily system
– MS type	BDS subtype characterised by musculoskeletal tension and pain
– GI type	BDS subtype characterised by gastrointestinal symptoms
– GS type	BDS subtype characterised by general symptoms (fatigue, headache, etc.)
– CP type	BDS subtype characterised by cardiopulmonary symptoms
BDS, multi-organ type	The most severe form of BDS, characterised by symptoms from at least three bodily systems
CFS	Chronic Fatigue Syndrome
CMDQ	Common Mental Disorder Questionnaire
CNS	Central Nervous System

DSM-IV	Diagnostic and Statistical Manual of Mental Disorders, fourth edition
FIP-study	Functional Illness in Primary Care (A study of prevention and treatment of functional illness in primary care performed in Aarhus, Denmark)
f-MR	Functional Magnetic Resonance
GP	General practitioner
IBS	Irritable Bowel Syndrome
ICD-10	International Classification Diseases and Health Related Problems, tenth revision
ICPC	International Classification of Primary Care
MCS	Multiple Chemical Sensitivity
MUS	Medically Unexplained Symptoms
PET	Position Emission Tomography
SCAN	Schedules for Clinical Assessment in Neuro-psychiatry
STreSS	Specialised Treatment for Severe Bodily Distress Syndromes
TERM	The Extended Reattribution and Management Model
WHO	World Health Organization

PART I

INTRODUCTION TO
FUNCTIONAL DISORDERS

CHAPTER 1

Background

PER FINK, MARIANNE ROSENDAL, TOMAS TOFT AND ANDREAS SCHRÖDER

The essential characteristics of functional disorders are that the patient is troubled by physical symptoms that cannot be attributed to any known, well-defined physical or psychiatric disorder, i.e. functional or medically unexplained symptoms. In the International Classification of Primary Care (ICPC) [12], the ICD-10 and the DSM-IV, functional disorders are classified mainly under the subgroup of somatoform disorders (P75/F45.0-9). Usually included within this category of functional disorders are the dissociative disorders (P75/F44.0-9), neurasthenia (P78/F48.0), factitious disorder, including Münchhausen's syndrome (P80/F68.1) and elaboration of physical symptoms for psychological reasons (P80/F68.0). The somatoform diagnoses have never been widely accepted outside of psychiatry and are rarely used by non-psychiatrists.

Various medical specialties have instead introduced a number of so-called functional syndrome diagnoses (see Table 1.1), which largely reflect the same phenomenon. Like the somatoform disorders, these syndrome diagnoses are based solely on subjective complaints and not on verifiable clinical or paraclinical findings, and the cause of the symptoms is unknown. Clinically, it is difficult to distinguish them from each other or from the somatoform disorders since the diagnostic criteria overlap and the patients are presenting the same symptoms [13-21]. The syndromes may therefore partly be seen as artificially created variants of functional disorders that arise owing to the medical specialisation, where each medical specialty has introduced its own diagnosis of medically unexplained symptoms [14-17;21]. Which diagnosis the patients receive sometimes depends more on what specialty they are referred to, or on the respective doctor's interest, than on which symptoms they actually have.

Table 1.1 Functional somatic syndromes according to specialty. Modified after Wessely [14;29]

Specialty	Functional somatic syndrome
Allergy and others	Multiple chemical sensitivity (MCS), sick building syndrome) hypersensibility to electricity, hypersensibility to infrasound
Anaesthesiology	Chronic benign pain syndrome
Gastroenterology	Irritable bowel syndrome (IBS), non-ulcer dyspepsia
Gynaecology	Pelvic girdle pain, premenstrual syndrome (PMS), chronic pelvic pain
Infectious medicine	Chronic fatigue syndrome (CFS, ME)
Cardiology	Atypical or non-cardiac chest pain, syndrome-X
Respiratory medicine	Hyperventilation syndrome
Neurology	Tension headache, pseudo-epileptic seizure
Odontology	Temporomandibular joint dysfunction, atypical facial pain
Orthopaedic surgery	Whiplash-associated disorder (WAD)
Psychiatry	Somatoform disorders, neurasthenia, conversion disorder
Rheumatology	Fibromyalgia, lower back pain
Ear, nose and throat	Globus sensation, vertigo, tinnitus

Recent research has shown that patients can be divided into two groups: one group who has symptoms from multiple organ systems, and another group who predominantly has symptoms from a single organ system (e.g. a musculoskeletal type identical with fibromyalgia; see Figure 1.1).

Thus, subtypes of functional disorders can be defined by symptom patterns. All patients typically have multiple symptoms simultaneously as an expression of bodily distress, and the disorder is therefore termed *bodily distress syndrome* (see pages 27-8). The syndromes in Table 1.1 are best understood as an expression of bodily stress and not as classical physical diseases, which is supported by the fact that psychological therapies and drugs acting on the CNS (antidepressants, antiepileptics) have proven effective; inversely, it has not been possible to demonstrate the efficacy of medical or

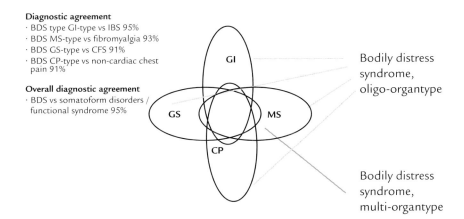

Diagnostic agreement
· BDS type GI-type vs IBS 95%
· BDS MS-type vs fibromyalgia 93%
· BDS GS-type vs CFS 91%
· BDS CP-type vs non-cardiac chest
  pain 91%

Overall diagnostic agreement
· BDS vs somatoform disorders /
  functional syndrome 95%

GI

GS   MS

CP

Bodily distress
syndrome,
oligo-organtype

Bodily distress
syndrome,
multi-organtype

Figure 1.1 **A theoretical model of BDS and empirical diagnostic agreement of its subtypes with existing diagnostic categories according to a Danish study [21]**. The percentages show how many patients who at the same time were either diagnosed with both a BDS subtype and the corresponding functional syndrome, or diagnosed with none of these. The remaining patients – e.g. 5% in connection with the BDS-GI subtype – were either diagnosed with only the BDS subtype or with the functional syndrome.
CFS: chronic fatigue syndrome; CP: cardiopulmonary; GI: gastrointestinal; GS: general symptoms; IBS: irritable bowel syndrome; MS: musculoskeletal. [21-23].

surgical treatment [23-26] directed against a hypothetical, presumed causes, such as antibiotics or immuno-suppressants for chronic fatigue syndrome or a stiff neck collar for WAD. Hence, today there is a significant linguistic and conceptual confusion in this area, and a host of other names for functional disorders have been or are currently being used [27;28].

Terminology used

The main terms currently used are *medically unexplained symptoms* (MUS) and *functional symptoms and disorders*. The term 'medically unexplained' has the disadvantage of indicating that the phenomenon is an exclusion diagnosis, used only when all physical diseases that may cause the symptoms have been excluded. Furthermore, modern scanning techniques and biophysiological measurements suggest the existence of a neurophysiological and biological basis for functional disorders and therefore indicating that the term be misleading [29;30].

The term *functional disorders* has been used over the past 150 years, especially in neurology. The term *functional* traditionally refers to reversible functional disturbances in the organ function, which were historically seen as a contrast to the irreversible structural pathoanatomical changes. In recent literature, the term is most often used to describe disorders of symptom perception and symptom production, i.e. dysfunction primarily located in the central nervous system [30].

Recently, the term *bodily distress disorder or syndrome* and, similarly, *bodily distress* designating the physical symptoms, have been coined [19;21] as neutral terms.

Health anxiety is characterised by the patient being excessively worried about his or her health and tormented by illness thoughts that are hard to stop. In the ICD-10 and the DSM-IV, the diagnosis used carries the older name hypochondria. There is no international consensus on which terms should be used, but bodily distress syndrome and functional disorder come out as the favourites in international research [30].

We will predominantly use the terms functional symptoms and disorders and bodily distress syndrome, as these terms are the most comprehensive and neutral in relation to the patient [31].

Definitions

+ **Functional symptoms** can be defined as symptoms caused by disturbances in symptom perception and/or symptom production, e.g. due to the arousal with hyperactivity in the autonomic nervous system. The symptoms are not better explained by another, traditionally defined physical disease or psychiatric illness.
+ **Functional disorders:** Disorders where the individual is experiencing physical symptoms affecting the daily functioning or quality of life, and where the symptoms cannot be explained better by any other physical disease or psychiatric disorder, or conditions where the individual is excessively worried about his or her health.
+ **Functional somatic** syndromes is a term used for syndromes defined solely by the patient's subjective complaints, and where no signs or paraclinical findings support the diagnosis. Their cause is unknown, but the name often carries a hypothetical presumption of a causal relationship. The concept of functional disorders includes functional somatic syndromes.

CHAPTER 2

Prevalence

PER FINK, MARIANNE ROSENDAL, TOMAS TOFT AND ANDREAS SCHRÖDER

Prevalence of physical symptoms

Population studies have shown that most people have daily bodily sensations or symptoms. A Danish study found that within the past two weeks, 84% of women and 75% of men had experienced at least one of the 13 specified symptoms [31]. The study found a slight decrease in symptom frequency with age. 47% of the women and 32% of the men indicated that they had been very troubled by their symptoms (Figure 2.1) [32].

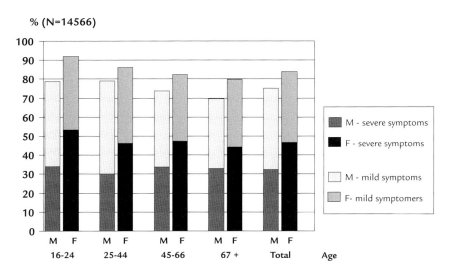

Figure 2.1 Two-week prevalence of physical symptoms among the general Danish population distributed on males (M) and females (F)[32]

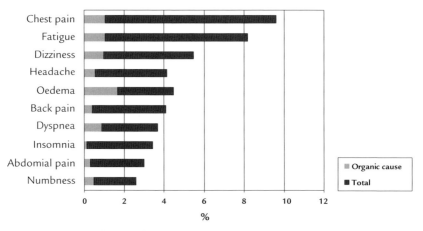

Figure 2.2. Diagnosed physical disease in 18-64 year olds after 3 years of follow-up [33]

An American study of the 25 most common physical symptoms among patients who sought medical treatment found that the cause of a diagnosable physical disease was found in only 10-15% of the cases after 3 years of follow-up (Figure 2.2 [33]).

It is thus more the exception than the rule that a physical symptom can be explained by a known physical disease. It may therefore be difficult to determine a precise boundary between what is normal and that which demands treatment. The frequency of functional disorders in the population is not precisely known because population studies have shown large differences in prevalence rates which range from 1% to 19% [34]. A large meta-analysis of population studies found a prevalence of ICD-10 somatoform disorders of 6.3%, which was almost identical to the frequency of depression of 6.9% [35]. Studies using standardised psychiatric interviews have shown that 20-30% of consecutive patients admitted to general hospital wards, or contact a general practitioner have an actual mental disorder [36-41].

The most frequent mental disorders in primary care are somatoform disorders, depressive disorders and anxiety disorders [36;37;42-47]. There is a substantial comorbidity between these disorders. For somatoform disorders, it has thus been shown that about 50% of the patients also suffer from another mental disorder, notably depression and anxiety [38;48].

Prevalence of functional disorders

Table 2.1 lists the prevalence of functional disorders of different clinical populations by selected ICD-10 diagnoses. It appears that about 25% of the patients who consult their general practitioner or are admitted to a general hospital unit suffer from a somatoform disorder, according to the ICD-10 criteria, and when consulting their general practitioner many present physical symptoms without a verifiable organic basis [42]. General practitioners estimate that the functional somatic symptoms play a significant role in 10-15% of the consultations by adults in primary care [49;50].

Table 2.1 Prevalence of functional disorders. Selected diagnoses.

Diagnosis	General Practice * %	Medical department ** %	Neurological department *** %
At least one functional somatic symptom	59-61	47	70
Somatoform disorders, total	**22-36**	**18-20**	**34**
Somatisation disorder	1-10	2-5	1-4
Somatoform pain disorder	4-10	2	10-11
Chronic fatigue syndrome (neurasthenia)	4	6	2
Hypochondria (health anxiety)	1-10	4-5	1-2
Dissociative disorder	0-4	2	2-3

*[38,42,51-55]; **[56]; ***[57].

According to several population studies, it is estimated that chronic fatigue occurs in up to 3% of the population, fibromyalgia in 1-11% and irritable bowel syndrome in approximately 7-22% [58-64]. A study in primary care, a department of internal medicine and a department of neurology, reported a prevalence of 3.7% for fibromyalgia, 2.9% for chronic fatigue syndrome, 2.8% for irritable bowel syndrome, 7.7% for chest pain, 2.6% for hyperventilation syndrome and 8.6% for pain syndrome [21].

Bodily distress syndrome

Seen from a more modern approach, functional disorders are comprised primarily of two main groups: *bodily distress syndrome* and health anxiety. These diseases are described on pages 27-8 and 31-2. A recent study showed that the prevalence of severe or multi-organ type *bodily distress syndrome* was higher among women (4.7%) than among men (1.2%), but it was independent of age [19]. The prevalence was similar among neurological, medical and primary care patients. The prevalence of moderate or single organ system *bodily distress syndrome* was 25.3% (women 28.6%, men 20.4%), and it was highest among patients under 65 and among neurological and primary care patients compared with medical patients. All studies show that women are over-represented among patients with functional disorders with physical symptoms by a factor of 2-6. Functional or somatoform disorders often have an onset before the age of 30-40 years. The prevalence according to age distribution is probably fairly constant. In difficult cases, the disease is often protracted, but with significant fluctuations in intensity. The disease may in some cases remit spontaneously.

Health anxiety

The other main group within the functional spectrum is constituted by health anxiety. It is shown that 1-2% of the population suffers from health anxiety or hypochondria according to the ICD-10-and the DSM-IV criteria, and the prevalence among those seeking medical attention is 1-10% [34;42]. A study showed that 9.5% of 18-65-year olds who consulted their general practitioner to discuss a new health problem suffered from health anxiety [51]. Health anxiety is equally frequent among men and women and independent of age. The disorder is not associated with education, marital or other socioeconomic factors [51]. In a study where patients were followed over a 2-year period after having visited their general practitioner, it was shown that patients were likely to continue being plagued by their health anxiety, and these patients had a high use of health services [65]. In severe cases, the disorder may lead to disability, but generally, the disease is less debilitating than *bodily distress syndrome*.

Consumption of health and social services

Patients with functional disorders have a high use of health services, both in primary care and in the specialised healthcare. In severe cases, the patient may over time have gone through numerous hospitalisations, surgery and futile treatment attempts and may have been inflicted with iatrogenic harm due to the many procedures [17;66]. Functional disorders account for at least 10-15% of the cases awarded early retirement in Denmark [67]. Since functional disorders often have an onset in a young age, such disorders may lead to the loss of working years and to a high cost of pension and social benefits.

Symptoms and symptom patterns described in patients with functional disorders have varied much throughout history and have been strongly influenced by the sociocultural context and the diagnoses which are "in vogue" [28]. It is therefore uncertain whether the prevalence of functional disorders has increased over time as we may attribute the apparent differences in prevalence to changes in the diagnostic terms deployed at various times in history. No certain differences in prevalence between different countries and cultures have been reported [46].

We may hence conclude that functional disorders are frequent in all parts of the healthcare system, and they are associated with significant costs and expenses, not only for society, but also for the individual patient in terms of the suffering they incur.

Summary

+ Physical symptoms with no known organic cause are common.
+ There is a high comorbidity between functional disorders, depression and anxiety disorders.
+ It is rather the exception than the rule that a specific organic disease is found in patients seeking medical advice because of bodily symptoms.
+ Population studies have found a prevalence of 6% for somatoform disorders. In clinical populations, severe bodily distress syndrome is reported to have a prevalence of 4.7% among women and 1.2% among men.
+ The prevalence of health anxiety is 1-2% within the general population and 5-9% in primary care.
+ The prevalence of somatoform disorders in primary care is 20-30%.
+ 10-15% of cases of awarded disability pension in Denmark, may be ascribed to functional disorders.
+ There are no documented differences in prevalences of functional disorders reported for different countries and cultures.

CHAPTER 3

Symptoms, clinical findings and the diagnostic process

PER FINK, MARIANNE ROSENDAL AND TOMAS TOFT

Classification and definition

As stated in the previous chapter, most people have daily bodily sensations, and it is more the exception than the rule that these sensations can be explained by a physical disease [33]. Bodily sensations are therefore considered part of the human sensory system whose task it is to monitor the body's functions and send a message to the person, when attention is needed. We also get bodily sensations when we sharpen our attention on the body or become frightened, and the sensation is not in itself an indication of pathology. A sensation acquires *clinical relevance* only when an individual or a doctor thinks that it can be a sign of an illness, in which case they are referred to as symptoms (Table 3.1).

With the exception of pathognomic findings, symptoms and findings are not conclusive, but need further modification to become meaningful in a clinical context. When the patient for example complains about having chest pain, this is hardly very informative or *specific* information because many different causes of chest pain exist. A *specification* or *precise description* of the symptom is therefore required; specifying, for example, whether the pain is retrosternally localised, is of a stabbing or pressing nature, its

Table 3.1 Classification of symptoms and clinical findings

Symptoms can be divided into:
- **Subjective symptoms**, which are sensations and other complaints that cannot be verified by any other person or by available examinations like for example pain and paraesthesia.
- **Objective sympt**oms, which are the patient's observations of his/her body and its secretions, e.g. haematuria and icterus, and the observations made by others than the therapist. Contrary to subjective symptoms, objective symptoms can be verified.

Clinical findings made during the clinical examination may be divided into:
- **Provoked findings**, i.e. subjective symptoms like soreness resulting from pressure or sensory impairment unnoticed by the patient until objective physical examination.
- **Certain find**ings, which may be objective symptoms that are verified or phenomena unnoticed by the patient such as abdominal mass or cardiac murmur.

Pathognomic findings are defined as:
- Findings on which a certain diagnosis can be made, for example fractured bone visible in a wound would suffice to make a diagnosis of open fracture.

strength, variation over time, if it is radiating, its chronology, accompanying symptoms, and whether there are triggering/soothing factors. Such specification is required for the doctor to be able to *classify* the complaint within a named *category* using a particular *technical term*, such as angina pectoris. A collection of symptoms that often occur simultaneously or are mutually related is called a *syndrome* [68]. Medical thinking assumes that such symptoms overlap because they have a common biological origin. The cause may be known like in angina pectoris or unknown like in rheumatoid arthritis. The diagnosis represents the highest level of abstraction. Besides symptomatology, clinical and paraclinical findings, the concept of diagnosis embraces also knowledge of causal factors, course and treatment.

Common symptoms of stress and strain

Analyses of symptom patterns have shown that humans, when exposed to stress and strain, have some general reaction patterns. These can be roughly divided into three main types, namely, bodily reactions, emotional reactions and cognitive reactions (Figure 3.1). Some symptoms are so general and unspecific that it is debatable whether they should be classified as physical, emotional or cognitive symptoms. These include e.g. fatigue,

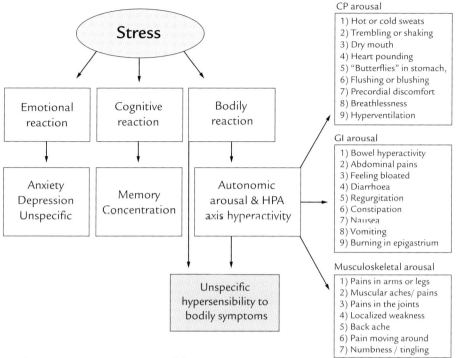

Figure 3.1 Latent structure model

sleep disturbances and headaches, which occur in a variety of illnesses as well as in healthy subjects.

Physical symptoms

All studies unanimously report that patients who are exposed to stress are likely to report *many symptoms*, i.e. they have a diffuse, reduced threshold for registering or reporting symptoms. An analysis of physical complaints that cannot be attributed to any known physical disease has established the symptom groups featured in Table 3.2 [19;69]. These symptom patterns can probably be attributed to central processes. The cardiopulmonary or autonomic symptom group is well-described and can be attributed to an activation of the sympathetic autonomic nervous system. This symptom group is also called *arousal* symptoms. The symptoms are frequent in anxiety. The gastrointestinal symptoms can probably be attributed to the parasympathetic autonomic nervous system and the activation of formatio reticularis in the brain stem by symptoms emanating from the musculoskeletal/loco-motor system. All these groups are therefore subject to regulation by the hypothalamus or regulation from a higher level in the CNS. The HPA axis with the stress hormones adrenaline and cortisol are likely to be involved (as a mediating mechanism). However, the central mechanisms and their physiology are inadequately explored, and other mechanisms may also be involved (see also Chapter 6).

Table 3.2 Common physical reactions to stress and strain. The symptom patterns are based on a statistical analysis of 972 psychiatric interviews (SCAN) [19].

Cardiopulmonary/ autonomic arousal	Gastrointestinal arousal	Muscles/joints and sensory Disturbances	General symptoms
Hot or cold sweats	Frequent loose bowel movements	Pain in arms or legs	Concentration difficulty
Trembling or shaking	Abdominal pain	Muscular aches and pains	Excessive fatigue
Dry mouth	Feeling bloated / full of gas / distended	Pains in the joints	Tension headache
Palpitations	Diarrhoea	Feeling of paresis or localised weakness	Impairment of memory
Churning in stomach, "butterflies"	Regurgitation	Backache	Dizziness
Flushing or blushing	Constipation	Pain moving	
Precordial discomfort	Nausea	Unpleasant numbness or tingling sensations	
Breathlessness without exertion	Vomiting		
Hyperventilation	Burning sensation in chest or epigastrium		

Emotional symptoms

The emotional reactions can be divided into depressive symptoms and anxiety/nervous symptoms (Table 3.3). These types of reactions also include sleep disorders like difficulty falling asleep, interrupted sleep, early morning awakening and being insufficiently rested when waking up, etc.

Table 3.3 Common emotional reactions to stress and strain. The symptom patterns are based on a statistical analysis of 978 psychiatric interviews (SCAN) [19].

Depressive reaction	Nervous reaction
Depression	Worry-prone
Tearfulness	Restlessness / inner uneasiness
Isolation tendency	Tiredness
Reduced interest/enjoyment	Sensitivity to noise
Feeling of guilt	Irritability
Reduced self-confidence	Tense and feeling of being under pressure
Hopelessness about the future	Muscular tension
Thoughts about suicide or death	Tension ache (e.g. headache, back ache)

Cognitive symptoms

Finally, cognitive symptoms are common in strain and stress, just as they are frequent in various psychiatric disorders (Table 3.4). Table 3.4 also includes *subjective memory difficulties,* i.e. memory problems that cannot be verified by neuropsychological or other testing methods.

Table 3.4 Common cognitive reactions to stress and strain.

Concentration difficulty

Memory impairment*

Difficulty thinking clearly and making decisions

Loss of interest

Loss of energy

Becomes overwhelmed by everyday tasks

The symptom patterns are based on a statistical analysis of 978 psychiatric interviews (SCAN) [19].
* The inclusion of this symptom, which was not part of the analysis, is warranted by clinical experience.

How to make a diagnosis
What is demanded of a diagnosis?

Several criteria must be met in order to establish a diagnosis based on symptoms. Kendell established [70] a number of strategies to validate clinical syndromes and diagnoses. The first step is to identify a characteristic symptom pattern. The next strategy is to investigate whether a suspected syndrome may be distinguished from other similar syndromes. Such demarcations have neither been established for the somatoform diagnoses in the ICD-10 and the DSM-IV in general, nor for the functional syndromes (Table 1.1). Any distinction must necessarily be made on the basis of representative populations, but many diagnoses whose cause is unknown have been developed based on selected patient populations like patients referred to a highly specialised hospital ward. The other strategies deployed to validate clinical diagnoses include the demonstration of heredity in family and twin studies, characterisation of a unique course or prognosis, or identification of a specific response to therapy. The ultimate validity criterion, according to Kendell, is the detection of a more basic abnormality or mechanism to explain the disease, be it psychological, pathophysiological or pathoanatomical, i.e. demonstration of a secure and verifiable underlying cause.

Modern medicine is deeply rooted in the Hippocratic fundamental principle that the cause of a disease must be found, as only treatment directed at the cause is effective. The principle of investigating diseases has therefore been that one tries to correlate symptoms and symptom patterns to organ-pathology or to a pathophysiological mechanism in order to identify the underlying cause or mechanism behind the disease. This so-called machine error model has proven extremely effective, and today we have complete or partial knowledge of the cause of many physical diseases. Nevertheless, this success has meant that there is a tendency to forget the basic diagnostic principles stated by Kendell, although they are crucial in cases where the diagnosis is based on subjective symptoms and provoked clinical findings and not on verifiable clinical and paraclinical findings. A common error is the establishment of hypotheses about a suspected causal relationship without having ascertained that what is being analysed is actually a discrete, well-delineated syndrome. For example, many of the functional syndromes (see Table 1.1) have been named on the basis of a supposed causation, and they are often based on consensus, i.e. diagnostic criteria based on consensus among a number of prominent individuals within each scientific/clinical environment [61]. Hereby, the diagnostic approach becomes narrow because it is based on a limited patient population rather than describing syndromes according to Kendell's overarching principles.

Making a diagnosis in clinical practice

In clinical practice, the doctor seeks to make a diagnosis by establishing a correlation between the patient's symptoms, clinical and paraclinical findings, and a known disease picture. This process simultaneously excludes other differential diagnoses. This model has proven effective in diseases where the cause is known and the diagnosis is documented by means of verified clinical and paraclinical findings. The disadvantage of this method is that the doctor may focus on getting specific diagnoses confirmed by concentrating exclusively on symptoms confirming his or her hypothesis and ignoring symptoms pointing to a differential diagnosis. The diagnosis thus depends on the "eye of the beholder", i.e. the doctor's knowledge, skill, diligence, urgency and professional orientation. For example, a gynaecologist will firstly think of a gynaecological disease and may be inclined to ignore symptoms not belonging to his or her specialty. It is important in the diagnostic process that the doctor maintains a broad approach to the patient's symptom picture and avoids focusing on a particular diagnostic process from the beginning.

Summary

+ Strain or stress (whether physical or emotional) may lead to a diffusely reduced threshold for symptom registration
+ The general physical symptoms of stress and strain can be divided into: cardiopulmonary, gastrointestinal, musculoskeletal and general symptoms.
+ A person may also react to stress or strain with emotional or cognitive symptoms, and these symptoms can be divided into symptoms of depression, nervousness and cognitive impairment.

CHAPTER 4

Classification and characteristics

PER FINK, MARIANNE ROSENDAL AND TOMAS TOFT

Classification of patients with functional symptoms

The validity of the ICD-10-and the DSM-IV classification of somatoform disorders is highly critical because the individual diagnoses are arbitrarily defined and poorly delineated, which implies that patients will often meet the criteria for several diagnoses at the same time. Furthermore, according to the ICD-10, a somatoform diagnosis requires a disease duration of at least 6 months. Because physical symptoms are exceedingly common in the population, the phenomenon must be considered to span a spectrum from mild cases, which are difficult to distinguish from normal conditions, to severe, chronic cases. The mild cases cannot be classified according to the ICD-10, but are typically classified under the symptom diagnoses in the ICPC (International Classification of Primary Care).

In this book, we will use the classification of disorders with the physical symptoms as listed in Table 4.1 [71;72]. The classification also includes the milder and non-pathological cases (I, II and III). The latter may attract medical attention and may therefore be of differential diagnostic significance.

Included in the category of functional disorders are *bodily distress syndrome*, health anxiety, dissociative disorders with motor or sensory symptoms and *factitious disorder*, including Münchhausen's syndrome. The other disorders listed in Table 4.1 may in some cases only manifest themselves in emotional or behavioural symptoms.

Table 4.1 A framework for categorization of patients presenting with functional somatic symptoms in primary care. Modified according to Fink et al [72].

	Category	Clinical presentation
I.*	Symptom diagnoses: Mild and transient symptoms	No significant impact on functioning or well-being. Does not meet the criteria for either mental or physical disease. No indication for treatment, but avoid placing patient in sick role by unnecessary examinations and biomedical treatments.
II.*	Natural (dis)stress reaction	Natural reactions to life events like bereavement, loss of job, divorce, etc. The distress does not exceed what would be expected from exposure to the stressor. The person may complain of a wide range of unspecific physical, cognitive and emotional symptoms. Symptoms do not meet the criteria for a psychiatric disorder.
III.*	Distress/stress/strain/adaptation reactions With primary: i. Physical symptoms ii. Emotional symptoms iii. Mixed symptoms iv. Unspecific symptoms	The patient presents unspecific physical, cognitive, emotional or behavioural symptoms. Marked distress and significant impairment in social or occupational functioning and wellbeing. If exposed to identifiable stressor, the reaction exceeds what would be expected. The extent and characteristics of the disturbances do not meet the criteria for a more specific mental disorder (given its duration, symptom picture, severity, etc.). Treatment consists of general care and psychological counselling to support the patient in coping with and managing any stress and traumas. Medical treatment is rarely indicated.
IV	Bodily distress syndrome	The patient usually presents with multiple functional bodily symptoms (see Table 4.2, *bodily distress syndrome*). The symptoms are severe and persistent and markedly affect the patient's wellbeing and ability to function. Includes somatisation disorder, undifferentiated somatoform disorder, pain disorder, chronic fatigue syndrome, neurasthenia and other functional syndromes.

V	Health anxiety (including hypo-chondriasis)	Excessive and inappropriate worry and pre-occupation with having or getting a serious physical disease.
VI	Dissociative (conversion-) disorders	Pseudo-neurological symptoms, i.e. physical symptoms or deficits simulating neurological disorders such as paresis, blindness or amnesia. The onset is sudden and closely associated in time with identifiable, emotionally traumatic events, insoluble and serious problems or difficulties in relation to other people. The symptoms are not better accounted for by an identifiable physical disease or other mental disorder.
VII	Factitious disorder and Münchhausen's syndrome	Intentional self-inflicted disease or induction or pretention of physical symptoms without clear, external motive (e.g. economic gain or avoiding legal responsibility).
In connection with other disorders		
VIII	Physical symptom presentation in other mental disorder	Physical symptoms due, for example, to depression or anxiety disorder. The patient meets the criteria for having the core disorder, and the physical symptoms can be explained as manifestations of this core disorder.
IX	Psychological factors affecting a medical condition	Physical symptoms due to well-defined physical disease are aggravated and exacerbated.

I. Symptom diagnoses: Mild and transient symptoms

This group includes patients who consult their general practitioner due to trivial discomforts without any suspicion of disease and without the symptoms having a significant impact on their functioning and wellbeing. The patient only wants to be sure that he or she has no illness requiring treatment, or wants a health check, and the patient requests no treatment. It may not be entirely clear whether the patient has a mild form of a functional disorder or is just exhibiting normal behaviour. Prevention campaigns encourage the general population to get examined for the sake of early detection of cancer, hypertension, high cholesterol etc., and this behaviour may therefore be appropriate from a medical point of view. Many of the consultations in primary care fall into this category.

It is important that the doctor does not worry the patient unnecessarily, because of his/her medical uncertainty or because of a misguided openness about differential diagnostic considerations and the limitation of medical science with regard to excluding disease. The doctor should normalise the patient's discomfort and reassure the patient by drawing on the patient's own health beliefs. By multiple contacts, other diagnoses should be considered.

> **Example:** *A 22-year-old man who has had no previous major health problems contacts his general practitioner because of a lump in the groin. He is worried that it could be a tumour. At the physical examination, a lymph node of normal size is found. The patient is reassured that this is not something pathological, but a completely normal finding. The suspicion of cancer can thus be rejected. The patient leaves the surgery, happy and unworried and does not present with the same symptom again.*

II. Natural reactions to strain or stress

These reactions are natural reactions to psychological trauma or stress to which all people are exposed, e.g. bereavement, divorce, illness, job loss, etc. There is much difference in how people react to stress, and their emotional and physical reactions can be very violent without being pathological. The symptoms will often fall into the categories listed in Tables 3.1 to 3.3. If the actual response exceeds the expected response given the mental trauma, or if the person does not get over it again within a reasonable time, a mental disorder should be considered. With regard to the differential diagnosis of physical diseases, it is essential that the doctor is aware that stress reactions may take the form of physical symptoms. If the doctor is not aware of this and instead takes a narrow biomedical focus and makes unnecessary investigations and/or treatments attempts, the person may become medicalised. In people who are otherwise healthy, no treatment beyond ordinary care is required. It should be stressed, however, that any mental disorder should be treated, if possible, no matter what its cause is. There has been a growing tendency towards professionalising the management of natural reactions to stress, e.g. by referral to a psychologist. This is inappropriate, and resources seem better used for people who need professional help than for managing problems that are a natural part of human life. There is also the danger of neglecting the natural support of the social network as family and friends will not dare to step in because they are afraid not to be able to do as well as a professional.

> **Example:** *An elderly woman loses her adult son, who dies suddenly of a heart attack. She contacts the general practitioner because of shortness of breath and palpitations. She almost does not sleep at night because of a discomforting feeling that the heart beats too hard and sometimes also irregularly. She also occasionally gets a choking feeling during the night. After a few talks with her general practitioner, she gets an understanding of the natural grief she suffers because of her son's death, and she is informed about the physical symptoms of anxiety. The woman has a good network, which she is committed to use in a better way, and the symptoms subside as the grief is processed.*

III. Distress, stress and adjustment reactions

Distress or strain reactions include disorders and reactions that are more severe than normal, but do not have a severity or are of a nature meeting the criteria for severe mental illness or *bodily distress syndrome*. The patient complains of various unspecific nervous, physical, emotional or cognitive symptoms (see Tables 3.2 to 3.4). Symptoms from different organ systems often occur simultaneously, but symptoms from one domain can be dominant. The problem has a significant impact on the patient's social and occupational functioning or quality of life and is stronger than would be expected given the stress or the mental trauma suffered. The individual's predisposition and vulnerability play a significant role. Treatment consists of standard care and psychological counselling to facilitate the handling and processing of any stress and trauma. Medical treatment should only be used in exceptional cases.

> **Example:** *A female school teacher tells her general practitioner that she wants to be tested for "everything". She believes that something is very wrong with her. The woman herself thinks that either something is wrong with her immune system, that she is intolerant to certain kinds of food or some drugs, that something is wrong with the indoor environment at her workplace, or that she might have asthma. Her symptoms include fatigue, difficulty concentrating, shortness of breath, a feeling that she is shaking inside and a general feeling of being ill. It turns out that her symptoms get worse when she is at work and wear off when she is on vacation. After a few talks, it becomes clear that she has many conflicts with a class and that she has not felt supported by management. Via her employer, the woman is allocated 10 sessions with a psychologist to help her find ways of managing her working conditions. It is agreed with the management at the school that she should no longer have the class. The woman gets better.*

IV. Bodily Distress Syndrome (BDS)

The patient often presents a vague symptom picture with uncharacteristic and nonspecific physical symptoms, i.e. symptoms that are common in the population and in a wide variety of disorders (e.g., fatigue and headache). The patient typically complains of many symptoms, but their number may vary considerably from patient to patient and over time within the individual. Patients with a functional disorder may complain of any subjective physical symptoms and the symptoms may refer to any organ system. Patients may sometimes also complain about objective symptoms, e.g. by complaining about aggravation of symptoms associated with a physical disease and incorporation of these symptoms into their functional state. Similarly, positive clinical findings do not necessarily rule out the diagnosis. Congenital defects or degenerative lesions that are asymptomatic in most individuals may mistakenly be attributed clinical significance. The patient can, over time, have been exposed to multiple investigations, treatment attempts and invasive procedures, which may have resulted in organic complications. In chronic cases, the symptom picture may thus be a complex mixture of organic-based and medically unexplained symptoms and findings. The diagnostic criteria for bodily distress syndrome are listed in Table 4.2. The condition is categorised according to its duration into acute (2 weeks to 6 months), subacute (6 months to 2 years) and chronic (>2 years).

Table 4.2 Diagnostic criteria for *bodily distress syndrome*

Yes	No	Symptom group
		≥ 3 Cardiopulmonary/autonomic Palpitations/heart pounding, precordial discomfort, breathlessness without exertion, hyperventilation, hot or cold sweats, trembling or shaking, dry mouth, churning in stomach/"butterflies", flushing or blushing.
		≥ 3 Gastrointestinal symptoms Abdominal pains, frequent loose bowel movements, feeling bloated/full of gas/distended, regurgitations, constipation, diarrhoea, nausea, vomiting, burning sensation in chest or epigastrium.
		≥ 3 Musculoskeletal tension Pains in arms or leg, muscular pains or aches, pains in the joints, feelings of paresis or localised weakness, back ache, pain moving from one place to another, unpleasant numbness or tingling sensations.
		≥ 3 General symptoms Concentrating difficulties, impairment of memory, excessive fatigue, headache, dizziness.

1-2 yes: Moderate or single-organ system *bodily distress syndrome*.
3-4 yes: Severe or multi-organ system *bodily distress syndrome*.

Besides the symptom patterns listed in Table 4.2, a number of other characteristics may also be used in the diagnosis of more severe or chronic cases (Table 4.3).

The patient may find it difficult to clearly describe his or her symptoms, i.e. describe their intensity, quality and chronology. The discomfort experienced may be described as being of maximal intensity all the time, but if the doctor manages to make such patients keep a diary of symptom intensity, it will become clear that there is variation in intensity, from day to day and from year to year. The patient has difficulty in identifying factors relieving or aggravating the symptoms or the symptoms are numerous and diffuse. Current symptoms and signs of previous illness episodes can be mixed together in a confusing and inconsistent manner, and information can at times even be contradictory. This stands in contrast to patients with a physical disease who are usually very accurate in describing their symptoms.

Comparison of information from various sources often shows that subjective complaints and objective impression and functioning diverge. Symptoms may be inconsistent with the anatomy and pathophysiology, e.g. muscle

Table 4.3. Characteristic differences between well-defined physical disease and functional disorders

	Functional disorder	Physical disease
Symptom description		
Location	Vague, diffuse, alternating	Well-defined, constant
Intensity	Vague, indistinctly defined intensity, few variations, often at maximum at all times	Well-defined changes and levels of intensity
Periodicity	Diffuse, difficult to define, are often denied	Typically well-defined periods with aggravation or improvement
Relieving or aggravating factors	Vague, indistinct, numerous	Well-defined, few
Number of symptoms	Numerous, vague	Few, well-defined, clearly described
The nature of symptoms	Unspecific	Specific
The character of the symptoms	Uncharacteristic	Characteristic
Symptoms causing medical help-seeking	Vague, difficult to identify	Can be identified and distinguished from comorbid symptoms
Other characteristics		
Treatment and medication	Effect difficult to evaluate, transitory	Level of effect well-defined
Previous treatments	Unclear what treatment the patient has undergone. Diagnostic tests are often interpreted as treatment	The patient can account for previous treatments

weakness, tactile disturbances and sensory disturbances that do not follow nerve innervation pathways. *Emotional discrepancies* may also exist, where, for example, the patient appears remarkably unaffected emotionally by his or her illness despite the fact that he/she presents severe symptoms that threaten the future quality of life. Or the patient is *affective and highly emotionally charged* in his or her way of describing discomforts and the disease, i.e. they describe their situations in vivid, strong terms. Patients with severe functional disorders may focus on the suffering caused by their symptoms and on the negative impact the disease has on their lives and quality of life. Contrary to this, patients with well-defined physical diseases are more worried about the implications that their illness has on their future health, such as whether they will be healthy again, if it is something they can die from, etc. This so-called *emotional or psycho-social form of communication* in patients with functional disorders can put a significant pressure on doctors to "do something".

Patients with functional disorders can attribute their symptoms to a physical disease, and may in some cases be very persistent and unwilling or very reluctant to accept that they are not ill in any way that requires medical or surgical treatment. Most patients, however, are themselves in doubt about the cause of their illness and often have several explanatory models [73;74]. Whether the patient "has been persuaded" that the physical symptoms are due, for example, to stress and strain, or not, he/she may still be severely burdened by severe symptoms and therefore have a medical need for treatment. In severe cases, the patient can stage a fight to have his/her disorder recognised as a physical disease or to obtain acceptance of a particular causal explanation, e.g. a whiplash trauma or hypersensibility to electric or chemical substances. The patient may also struggle to get disability pension or compensation, often more to obtain recognition of his or her suffering than to obtain economic benefit.

In some cases, the disease onset may be rather abrupt in connection with a trauma or a physical disease in a previously unremarkable and well-functioning person. Such cases could for example be a whiplash trauma, a fracture, an infectious disease, an acute intoxication, back ache or the like. The symptoms persist even if, from a medical perspective, the initial disorder has been treated, and the patient is well as judged from biomedical parameters. Instead, the disease worsens over time with dominant symptoms like those listed in Table 4.2. Our knowledge of such a sudden onset is limited.

Example: A middle-aged woman, a social and health care worker, contacts her general practitioner with suspicion of a urinary tract infection. The woman says that she constantly feels her bladder and that this sensation reaches her kidneys. It affects her intestines, so that she often has loose stools, feels bloated and gets stomach aches. She fears that either she has an inflammation of the bladder, kidneys or a narrowing of her urinary tract. She also has pain in the lower back and neck, headache and difficulty concentrating. She has been having neck pain since she was hit from behind by a car almost 10 years ago. The woman believes that she has a whiplash injury that has never been recognized and for which she has never been compensated. She had to stop working 5 years ago due to pain in her arms, shoulders, legs and back. She now works part time in her spouse's company. This is not easy for her as they have many conflicts, and her spouse has difficulty understanding how she feels. Some days she has terrible pain throughout her body, and sometimes she is so tired that she can hardly stand upright, and she'll have to lie down. She is having a hard time relaxing because she constantly feels her heart when she is quiet. When she is well, she is trying to get as much done as possible. She has been thoroughly assessed in terms of orthopaedics, cardiology, neurology and gastroenterology, with no signs of disease in any of these organs. She has spent much money over time on physical therapy, chiropractic and various forms of natural medicine and alternative medicine. Most of this has had only temporary effect. She would now like her general practitioner to start a process of urological assessment and would like to have her kidneys scanned because she does not believe that they have ever been properly investigated. She believes that because she feels so ill, she must have an illness the doctors just have not yet found.

V. Health anxiety

Health anxiety is characterised by the patient's excessive worry about physical disease or the risk of contracting a disease. Awareness of and concern about one's health spans a spectrum ranging from something we all recognize to disorders where the patient is deeply concerned and crippled by his or her fear. We refer to health anxiety when the disorder is bothersome to the person and leads to a deterioration in the quality of life and functional capacity.

In the ICD-10 and the DSM-IV, the diagnosis used is hypochondria. The use of the word hypochondria is perceived by many as stigmatising, so the term health anxiety is preferred. Table 4.4 features the new, empirically validated diagnostic criteria for health anxiety [51]. It should be noted, however, that these new criteria have not been verified at any larger scale and they should therefore be considered with some caution.

The main symptom of health anxiety is *obsessive rumination* and thoughts or ideas about suffering from a disease (Table 4.4). When a patient first comes to think of a disease, he/she does not, or only with great difficulty, escape or stop thinking about this again. The thoughts centre on a suspected disease, and the patient can find more and more "evidence" that he/she suffers from an often severe disease. The growing anxiety spiral ultimately makes the patient seek medical attention.

The patient is *excessively preoccupied with disease and conscious of bodily sensations and body functions* as well as anything that may appear to be a sign of a pathological condition. The patient may display autonomic hypersensibility, hearing his/her own pulse or being aware of other natural physical phenomena of which others are rarely conscious. The patient may misinterpret these natural sensations and may develop ideas that it is something unnatural or sickly. For example, if the patient gets a bruise or irritated skin, he/she will be worried that it may be a sign of a serious undetected illness. The patient is inclined to choose the worst possible explanation, and a trivial disorder may be misinterpreted as being a serious ailment. The patient may also keep a close eye on bodily functions and inspect the body's waste products and secretions, and, for example, frequently measure body temperature and blood pressure. Patients with health anxiety have a significant *suggestive* or *autosuggestive* potential. If the patient hears or reads about a disease, he/she is inclined to fear having that disease. Likewise, if someone in the family, among friends, acquaintances or work colleagues gets ill, the patient may feel or fear to have the disease. It is likely that the patient may also fear becoming infected with a disease if he/she has been with an ill person, or if the patient touches dirty things or things that could be infected, such as a toilet seat.

Table 4.4 Criteria for health anxiety according to Fink et al [51]

A		Obsessive rumination with (intrusive) thoughts, ideas or fears of harbouring an illness that cannot be stopped or can be stopped only with great difficulty.
B		One or more of the following five symptoms
	1	a and/or b a. Worrying about or preoccupation with fears of harbouring a severe physical disease or the idea that disease will be contracted in the future or preoccupation with other health concerns. b. Attention to and intense awareness of bodily functions, physical sensations, physiological reactions or minor bodily problems that are misinterpreted as a serious disease.
	2	Suggestibility and auto-suggestibility- if the patient hears or reads about a disease, he/she is inclined to fear that he/she has that disease.
	3	Excessive fascination with medical information.
	4	Unrealistic fear of being infected/contaminated by something eaten or touched (e.g. a person you have touched).
	5	Fear of taking prescribed medication.
C		If a medical condition is present, the patient's reaction clearly exceeds what would be expected from the medical condition alone.
D		The symptoms are not better explained by another psychiatric disorder
E		The symptoms should be present most of the time and persist for at least 2 weeks.
F		Specification: **Severe:** At least one of the symptoms in criteria A and B is severely disturbing or significantly interferes with everyday activities. **Mild:** All others.

A patient with health anxiety may have an *exaggerated fascination with medical information*. The patient is preoccupied with health and information about disease in newspaper articles, magazines, popular medical books and television programmes and can be a frequent user of the Internet, etc. Because of a raised level of susceptibility and suggestibility, this interest may in some cases be a significant burden for the patient. In recognition of this, he/she may avoid dealing with health matters and fail to visit family members or friends who are hospitalized or ill, because it is so anxiety-provoking. The patient is often afraid to take *medication*.

> **Example:** *A man in his 50s is growing increasingly worried that he is seriously ill. He is especially worried that he is suffering from cancer and fears that it will not be detected in time. He begins to visit his general practitioner ever more often with mainly non-specific skin changes. The man will not be reassured that the general practitioner believes that the skin lesions are benign. He begins to seek information online and gets severe symptoms when he accidentally hears about illness. The man begins to withdraw from social interactions with friends and family, as he does not feel that they take him seriously. He has always had a tendency to worry about his health, but it has become much worse after a man of the same age living in the neighbourhood suddenly died of leukaemia.*

VI. Dissociative disorders

Dissociative (or *conversion*) *disorders* are disorders in which the patient presents (pseudo)neurological symptoms, i.e. symptoms simulating a neurological disorder, but the patient does not have a neurological disease. Symptoms may consist of paresis, sensitivity disturbances, cramps, blindness or cognitive symptoms such as memory loss. The syndrome occurs suddenly as a result of what in the person's eye is perceived as severe psychological distress or trauma, such as a serious accident, fire, a sudden death or an unexpected revelation of a crime the patient himself or close relatives have committed. Transient dissociative reactions are probably frequent, and by disasters and greater psychological trauma, even mentally stable people may react with dissociative symptoms. In most cases, the medical history will, however, contain information that suggests that the person is mentally vulnerable. In most cases, the disorder is transient and the patient improves spontaneously without treatment, but the disorder may in some cases take a chronic course.

Example: *A shop owner who has been in conflict with the municipality for several years receives a letter that his business must close by the end of the next month. This happens in the middle of the busy season of his business. After discussing the situation with his staff, he goes to collect goods at the shop as usual. He then does not remember what happened and he is found walking around in the forest at night, incoherent and confused. It later turns out that he has tried to hang himself. He is hospitalized in a neurological section because of suspicion of epilepsy, but this is ruled out. He is then transferred to the psychiatric unit where he receives a diagnosis of dissociative fugue. In the course of three days, he gets better and is back to normal when discharged.*

VII. Factitious disorder and Münchhausen's syndrome

Disordo factitious (factitious means fake or simulated) implies deliberate imitation or even self-inflicted disease where the person's own role is denied. Unlike other functional disorders, the patient is conscious about his own role in the disease, even if this is denied and kept hidden from the doctor [75]. Factitious disorder differs from malingering in that no obvious motive explains the behaviour [76;77].

Disordo factitious can be divided into four different types according to its clinical symptom presentation [78]:

+ Fictional case history, e.g. the patient for instance reports to have had a seizure, although it is not the case.
+ Simulated symptoms such as hearing loss.
+ Manipulation with certain clinical signs or paraclinical tests, e.g. by dripping blood in a urine sample or by manipulating a thermometer.
+ Self-induced illness or injury, such as hypoglycaemia by injecting insulin, abscesses after the patient has used an infected needle causing infection or poisoning, manipulation with surgical scars or existing illness.

Münchhausen's syndrome is a subgroup of *disordo factitious*, which, apart from self-induced or simulated disease, is characterised by *pseudologia fantastica* where the patient tells untrue stories, often of a grandiose character and also about other matters than his medical history. Furthermore, the disease is characterised by *shopping-around* in the sense that the patient travels from hospital to hospital to be hospitalised. Admissions are often *dramatic or happen under unusual circumstances* [78]. The syndrome is rare, but its exact prevalence is unknown [17]. Even so, because of the extremely high use of hospitalisations and consultations, most doctors will still come into contact with this type of patient. The psychiatrically closely examined cases of Münchhausen's syndrome presently available suggest that the syndrome masks a severe personality disorder, and instances of psychotic outbreaks are frequently reported [78-82]. The prognosis is poor, and the disorder must be regarded as a chronic.

> **Example:** *A woman in her 40s with approx. 20 hospitalizations due to abscesses in the thighs. Because of suspected immune deficiency as the cause of the recurrent abscesses, she is eventually moved from the local hospital to a highly specialized university hospital. No signs of immunological defects or other diseases are found. Microscopy of material from an abscess discloses a pin-prick and foreign objects, and it becomes evident that the patient herself has caused the abscesses by inject-ing herself with an infected needle. She is confronted with this and not hospitalized again because of abscesses.*

VIII. Malingering

Malingering is usually not perceived as an expression of abnormal psycho-pathology, but more as a legal problem. However, malingering can be a differential diagnostic problem. The phenomenon is widespread and can be seen, for example, among children who do not want to go to school, or among young people who want to avoid military service. It may also be seen in an effort to obtain a pension or compensation. In malingering, there is an obvious motive for the behaviour which the person, however, given the nature of this problem, tries to keep hidden. This separates malingering from *disordo factitious*, where there is no such motive. The malinger will take cost-benefit considerations into account, i.e. the advantage of malin-gering should preferably exceed the cost of the sick role. Malingers rarely inflict disease or harm on themselves other than in connection with war in which case self-inflicted wounds and injuries are not uncommon. Patients with *factitious disordo* do not consider the costs and benefits, and their self-inflicted diseases can be life-threatening, just as there are no limits as to which procedures, actions and physical treatments they are willing to undergo [78-83]. Malingering should be borne in mind when the disease in question has a medico-legal dimension, in anti-social personality disorder, when there is a discrepancy between objective findings and complaints, and when the person is uncooperative.

IX. Physical symptoms and illness worries in other mental disorders

Physical symptoms are prominent in many mental disorders and included in the diagnostic criteria of, for example, anxiety and depressive disorders. In most non-psychotic mental disorders, the patient mainly presents somatic and not emotional symptoms. This is true in 50-90% cases of depression and anxiety disorder [46]. This phenomenon has been referred to as presenting or facultative somatisation [53], but the terms do not seem well-chosen. There is nothing unnatural in fearing that you are suffering from a physical disease. The problem arises only if the doctor makes a wrong diagnosis, i.e. if it is the doctor rather than the patient who somatises. The typical clinical picture of a mental disorder will emerge when the history is taken, and the patient will usually accept the diagnosis when the correct diagnosis is made. The physical symptoms associated with depression or anxiety disorders occur simultaneously with the emotional and cognitive symptoms that characterise suffering. If it is possible to identify incidents of physical complaints that are independent of, for example, a depressive episode or a panic attack, two independent comorbid disorders should be considered. In severe depressive disorders, health worries are frequent, but in contrast to health anxiety, they will congruent with the patient's mood, i.e. they will bear the mark of the patient's depressive and pessimistic outlook. The physical symptoms and complaints will disappear when the mental disorder is treated.

> **Example:** *A man in his 40s contacts his general practitioner because of abdominal pain, which has lasted for about six months. The pain is non-specific and of varying intensity. His stools have not changed, but his appetite is reduced and he has lost around 4 kg. While taking his medical history, the practitioner discovers that over the past year he has also become ever more sad and prickly, his wife and children have begun to complain that he gets annoyed and irritable easily. He is tired during the day and sleeps poorly at night. He has gradually lost all his desire for sex. He thinks that he is a bad father and a bad husband, and that the family would probably be better off without him. In the course of the consultation, he is very close to tears, and when confronted with a direct question, he confesses that he has bought a rope and found the place where he would hang himself if he does not get better soon. Relevant tests for abdominal pain are taken and the man is treated for depression, after which his stomach pain goes away.*

X. Psychological factors affecting a medical condition

A patient in this group has a verifiable, well-defined physical disease, but there is a discrepancy between his subjective problems, his concerns, functional ability, treatment effect and severity of the disease as judged from the biomedical data. It can often be difficult to determine whether a patient is better classified under the group of functional disorders, because he may have incorporated his genuine physical disease into the functional disorder. In this case, it would also be inappropriate to make a sharp distinction between a mental disorder and a physical disease, as the problem is typically often both-and, especially in more chronic functional disorders.

> **Example:** *A woman in her 30s gets diagnosed with mild thyrotoxicosis. Receives medical treatment and reaches a reasonable level after some initial start-up problems. Still, she continues to consult her general practitioner quite often and would like to have her values checked because she thinks that she can feel that she is not sufficiently regulated. In some periods, she phones or sends an e-mail almost daily. She is very concerned about the disease, which she perceived as serious, and which, she feels, has grown out of proportions. She is acutely hospitalised a couple of times because she feels that her metabolism has gone completely wrong, but each time it turns out that her metabolism is entirely normal. The woman finds it ever more difficult to tend to her job as a teacher. She thinks that it is natural not to be able to work full-time when having a serious chronic disease.*

Diagnosis and differential diagnosis

The criteria stated in Tables 4.2 and 4.4 may be helpful in distinguishing diagnoses of functional disorders from diagnoses of physical diseases. Please note the presence of any current or previous psychiatric disorder; similarly, previous illness episodes of medically unexplained symptoms may support the diagnosis. It is, however, important to note that the diagnosis requires neither the presence of emotional symptoms, nor that any stress can be ascertained. The "nominal" value of the symptoms is of little differential diagnostic value, whereas non-specific or atypical symptoms, or a very unusual symptom presentation supports the diagnosis. Multiple fluctuating symptoms from many organ systems of unclear origin with a disease onset before the age of 30-35 years strongly support the diagnosis. On the other hand, physical and psychiatric differential diagnoses (depression, dementia, abstinence disorders) should be carefully excluded if a similar disease picture is seen in an older, formerly physically and mentally healthy patient.

A few well-defined physical diseases (hyperparathyroidism, hyperthyroidism, acute intermittent porphyria, myasthenia gravis, aids, multiple sclerosis, systemic lupus erythematosis, borrelia infection and connective tissue disorders) may present with many diffuse and non-specific symptoms from multiple body systems. In most of these diseases, positive clinical or paraclinical findings will verify the diagnosis. If one of these disorders is suspected, a *relevant test battery* may be to examine acute phase reactants (SR, CRP), renal function and electrolyte (sodium, potassium, creatinine, bicarbonate, calcium, phosphate), liver function (albumin, ALT, LDH, alkaline phosphatase and bilirubin), coagulation parameters (coagulation factors II, VII, X; APTT), haematologic status (haemoglobin, leukocytes, including differential count, platelets), vitamin deficiency (erypholate, p-cobalamin and vitamin D (S-25-OHD) endocrinological factors (TSH, glucose) and, possibly urine sticks. Depending on the symptomatology, also EBV antibodies, Borrelia serology and immunological parameters.

In well-defined physical diseases, the main symptoms are usually characteristic of the disease, i.e. they are the same from one patient to another and within the individual patient from one disease incident to another (see Table 4.3). Inversely, in functional disorders, the symptom picture is often not compatible with any known physical disease and it will fluctuate more over a period of time. Some physical diseases may also present with non-characteristic symptoms at onset, and we should be aware of the development of possible characteristic symptoms over time. It is extremely rare for major physical diseases to be overlooked among patients with functional disorders, but it should be remembered that a patient with a functional disorder may at the same time have or contract a physical disease. Instead of first eliminating even the rarest disease before considering a functional disorder, all differential diagnostic considerations should be included in the investigation from the very first contact with the patient in the same manner as when differential diagnostic considerations among various physical diseases are made.

Health anxiety is defined by its cognitive and emotional symptoms, whereas the physical complaints are not significant in themselves. The disease may occur simultaneously with *bodily distress syndrome* and with a physical disease. The diagnoses are not mutually exclusive. The dominant disease picture should primarily be diagnosed, but in some cases, it would be reasonable to apply both diagnoses.

Summary

- Functional disorders range within a spectrum from very mild cases, which are difficult to delimit against normal conditions, to severe chronic diseases.
- Functional somatic symptoms and disorders can be classified into different diagnostic categories, the most important of which are:
  a) *Natural reaction*: physical, emotional or cognitive symptoms in response to stress or strain.
  b) *Adjustment reactions*: physical, emotional or cognitive symptoms in response to changing terms of life; the reaction exceeds what is expected in the given situation.
  c) *Bodily distress syndrome*: severe functional disorder with symptoms from several organ systems.
  d) *Health* anxiety: excessive and undesirable worry and preoccupation or fear of having or developing a serious physical disease.

CHAPTER 5

Aetiology

PER FINK, MARIANNE ROSENDAL AND TOMAS TOFT

Causes

The aetiology of functional disorders, including that of functional syndromes, is only partially understood, but it is believed to be multifactorial, implying the interaction of biological, psychological and cultural (including political and administrative) factors as well as the healthcare system. Figure 5.1.A describes a matrix of the many factors involved. Furthermore, the time dimension of an illness course is illustrated in Figure 5.1 B. The illness processes are usually classified into *predisposing* factors (the person's susceptibility to develop the disease), *precipitating* (triggering) factors, which are those factors that directly cause the onset of the disease, and *perpetuating* (maintaining) factors which contribute to maintain or aggravate the patient's pathological processes. Early signs of disease are symptoms that are so discreet that the person and/or the doctor have not seen them as signs of disease, but retrospectively it may become evident that they were the first signs of the disease. This stage is followed by manifest disease and the rehabilitation phase, which can lead to one of the three final outcomes: recovery, chronic disability or death. At the heart of this overall disease model lies the observation that various aetiological and pathophysiological factors may be relevant at different times in the illness process, and it rarely makes sense to talk about "the cause". This is essential, in particular in functional disorders in which the predisposing and perpetuating factors seem to be particularly significant, whereas the triggers better determine *which* symptoms develop [84]. Even so, the patient (and the doctor) often

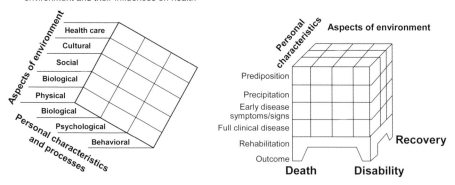

A Matrix for studying interactions of person and environment and their influences on health

B Phases of natural history of health illness continuum

Figure 5.1. A-B Multifactorial model of illness. Modified after Jenkins et al [85]

considers the triggers to be the "cause", e.g. a viral infection is the cause of chronic fatigue syndrome, even after the clinical virus infection is over. Or a traffic accident is considered the cause of the symptoms of chronic whiplash, although this cannot explain the persistence of the symptoms. Other possible causal explanations are thereby neglected.

Predisposing and precipitating factors

A number of non-specific *mental* and *social factors* may serve as *predisposing* factors in synergy with the person's general genetic and acquired susceptibility. Examples of non-specific factors could be the early loss of a close family member or a poor social background. These factors are called nonspecific, because they also make the individual susceptible to other ailments. Presumably more specific factors predisposing to functional disorders are physical or sexual abuse in childhood and one of the parents having had a functional disorder; by contrast, a well-defined physical disease in parents or child does not seem to predispose an individual to functional disorders. The family transmission may be rooted in socio-cultural learning, but much also suggests the presence of a moderate genetic susceptibility [48;86].

Functional disorders can be triggered by physical or psychological stress (precipitating factors) (Figure 5.2). These stressors can be physical, immunological, emotional or chemical, or there may be another mechanism by which the body's homeostasis is broken [87]. Examples include persistent symptoms after a whiplash trauma or chronic fatigue triggered by an infectious disease. This phenomenon has not been thoroughly studied, but one possible explanation is that the trauma/illness induces cerebral hypersensibility. Biological factors will be discussed in Chapter 6. Examples of emotional and social stressors may be the loss of a close relative, unemployment or financial problems.

Perpetuating factors

A *pathological cognitive processing* of information and physical sensations plays a role, both as a predisposing and a perpetuating factor. The cognitive processing will be reviewed in Chapter 8.

Social factors, including family circumstances, may be contributory factors, partly by imposing a mental strain on the patient, partly by keeping the patient in the sick role. In individual cases, financial aspects may work to enhance sustainability, e.g. if the patient is waiting to receive a pension or to receive claimed damages. In chronic fatigue syndrome, it has been shown that membership of a patient association/self-help group can be associated with a poor prognosis [88].

In addition to the patient or disease-related factors, the health care system or iatrogenic factors, i.e. the doctors' and the health care system's way of managing patients, may have an important bearing on the illness and its chronification. Doctors primarily tend to pursue organic explanations and only to a lesser extent other explanations, which may entail iatrogenic amplification of illness worry and illness behaviour [17]. The iatrogenic and social element is expressed in the broad definition of the overall somatisation concept, which has been proposed, among others, by the Canadian psychiatrist McDaniel: "A process whereby a doctor and/or a patient or family focuses exclusively and inappropriately on the somatic aspects of a complex problem" [89]. The iatrogenic factors will be discussed in Chapter 7.

The various aetiological factors play closely together, and even the biological factors must not be perceived as fixed; rather, they are subject to constant adaptation where new experiences are continuously validated and internalised within the individual. Moreover, the aetiology does not necessarily correlate with the treatment. The starting point of treatment also

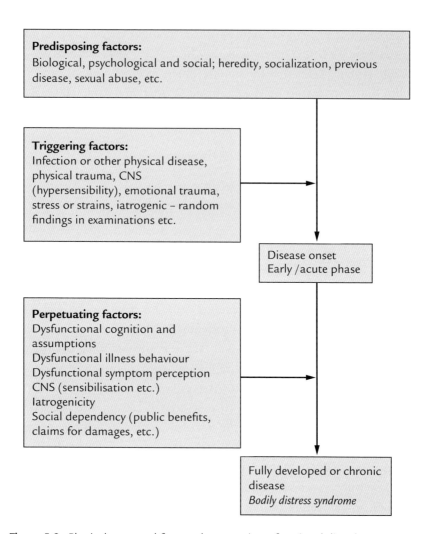

Figure 5.2. Physical or mental factors that can trigger functional disorders

depends on the range of available treatment modalities and expectations as to which treatment will be most efficient. It is not possible to draw up a simple model that includes the whole of this complexity, but the following chapters will review the most important elements.

Summary

+ The aetiology of functional disorders is partially unknown, but it is believed to be multifactorial.
+ The aetiological course can be divided into:
  - Predisposing factors such as heredity or social learning.
  - Precipitating factors such as trauma, stress or strain.
  - Perpetuating factors such as dysfunctional illness behaviour, or iatrogenic factors.

CHAPTER 6

Biological basis

PER FINK, MARIANNE ROSENDAL, TOMAS TOFT AND ANDREAS SCHRÖDER

Biological mechanisms

There is growing evidence that biological mechanisms are involved in functional disorders. On the one hand, a hereditary predisposition has been reported; on the other hand, a growing body of studies of functional somatic syndromes has shown changes in the brain function and even potential structural changes, and some studies have reported physiological changes [48, 87, 90-117]. Although there is currently little doubt that central mechanisms are involved, the results of neuroimaging (i.e. imaging techniques of the brain, such as PET and f-MRI) and pathophysiological studies have been disparate and sometimes in direct conflict with each other. Considerable uncertainty therefore prevails as to which mechanisms are actually involved. Based on empirical epidemiological studies, the prevailing hypotheses may be divided into two main groups: One group assumes the presence of a sensory dysfunction; the other assumes that symptoms are actively produced. The two types of hypotheses are not necessarily contradictory, but may be complementary (Table 6.1).

Table 6.1 Hypothesis of biological mechanisms of functional disorders

Pathological central processing and modulation of bodily stimuli

• Filter function
    – Myriads of bodily stimuli and sensations are constantly filtered in the brain, and normal people are conscious of only a small fraction of these stimuli.
• Hypersensibility, congenital or acquired, reinforces bodily stimuli
• Neural plasticity
    – Hypersensibilization
    – Prolonged activation
    – *Rerouting* of information from one region of the brain to another region that is normally not involved in this activity
• Transmitter imbalance
• Processing of bodily stimuli

Increased symptom production

• External stressors elicit bodily reactions/*arousal*
    – Activation of the autonomic nervous system, stress hormones and immune system
• Neural plasticity leads to
    – Hyperactivity
    – Prolonged activation
• Transmitter imbalance
    – Central nervous system defects that activate or does not suppress the autonomic nervous system and hormone system.

Pathological central processing and modulation of physical stimuli

The polysymptomatic illness picture in patients with a functional disorder may arise because the patient reinforces bodily sensations due to a central hypersensibilisation, or because afferent stimuli to the brain are not suppressed. Failure of suppression of afferent stimuli is referred to as an insufficient filtering function which implies that those sensations/symptoms that are normally being continuously evaluated at a subconscious level are suddenly invading the conscious mind [118]. This is the opposite of what can happen when a human is exposed to severe life-threatening stress, e.g. in a war situation or by an accident, where even very violent pain can be suppressed to ensure survival. Or the situation may be less dramatic as when the pain disappears from our consciousness when we become preoccupied with something else. Furthermore, via biological mechanisms, psychological factors may change perception thresholds, but there may also be a defect in

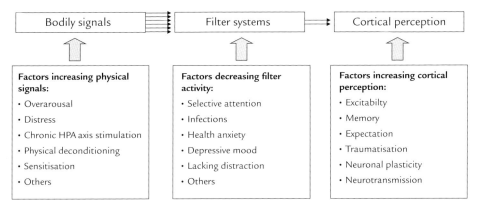

Figure 6.1 The filter model according to Rief et al [120]

the filter mechanism (see Figure 6.1). One study by James et al. [119] points to a fundamental neurophysiological disturbance in the attention process of patients with functional disorders. In studies with EEG monitoring of evoked potentials, they found that patients with functional disorders responded in the same manner to irrelevant and to relevant stimuli. In other words, patients with functional disorders do not filter out irrelevant stimuli.

Central sensibilisation is today a very widespread hypothesis in pain research [87, 99, 121-123]. Central *sensibilisation* incorporates a wide range of neurochemical and neurohormonal processes. The sensibilisation may be caused by prolonged stimulation or by stimulation of the somatosensory area in the brain, which then becomes hypertrophic or enhances sensibility in other ways. We may understand this in the same way as when a musician optimises the number and function of the neurons that have to do with finger motor function and sound perception. Similarly, persistent pain changes the neurons involved in the processing of pain stimuli. No matter how tempting the theory is, it does seem to be too simple, and the hypothesis is not supported by unanimous findings. For example, it has not been firmly established that pain thresholds are reduced in fibromyalgia; likewise, a higher pain threshold has been found in patients with many symptoms compared with healthy persons [98]. An explanation for this may, however, be that the hypersensibility is specific, so that sensitivity is only raised for certain pain modalities, whereas all other stimuli are suppressed or blocked, because the current pain dominates. It is also difficult to explain symptoms such as fatigue and paresis on the basis of a sensibilisation theory. The hypothesis also assumes the existence of a peripheral stimulus. We may, furthermore, hypothesise that the hypersensibility is of a more basic character, i.e. that it lies at a cellular, receptor or transmitter level.

A different, almost opposite hypothesis accepts the finding of a reduced sensitivity, i.e. an increased pain threshold, but this central hyposensibility is rooted in the inability or deficient fine-tuning of the complex network in the CNS to adequately process normal physical sensory stimuli. The person only reacts when the stimuli are sufficiently strong, and it may then be too late to prevent more pronounced or persistent discomforts. This may be another explanation for the higher pain threshold in patients with many symptoms [98]. Another study thus observed that patients with functional diseases found it much easier to lie still for a long period in PET scanners than normal control subjects. A wide range of different brain functions are involved in the sensory processing of physical sensory stimuli. Figure 6.3 illustrates the complex interplay in pain. Symptom processing may be disturbed by imbalances in the interaction between the different parts of the brain. One study found an increased pain threshold in patients with many symptoms. This finding was confirmed by pain simulation during PET scans, which found hypoactivity, but with activity in the same areas of the pain matrix as in normal subjects (see Figure 6.2) [98]. This imbalance means that the person experiences difficulty managing symptoms, which creates a pathological reaction when the capacity is exceeded. Individual elements of the sensory matrix may also be defectives and thereby cause suboptimal processing. Studies have indicated a dysfunction in the attention and in the secondary somatosensory area of the brain, as well as a hypersensibility of the limbic system to the physical stimuli in patients with functional disorders or syndromes [87,92,119,124-127]. The rough handling of stimuli may also be due to a transmitter imbalance.

Increased symptom production

The other main group of hypotheses argues that the CNS contributes to the production of symptoms. Encountering stress, physically and mentally, the body responds physiologically with an increased vigilance or a state of

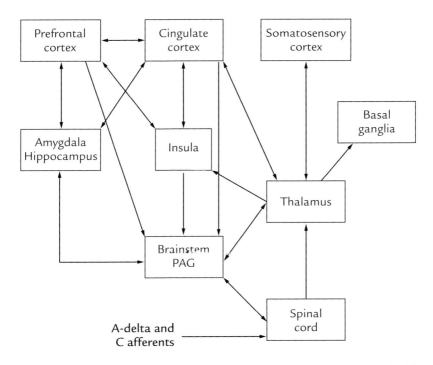

Figure 6.2 The pain matrix. The figure illustrates the many brain centres involved in the processing of pain and the complexity of the interplay between these centres [129].

alarm, also called the arousal. This arousal results in the production of a wide range of symptoms, as shown in Table 4.2, including a musculoskeletal arousal in the form of, inter alia, muscle tension. This activation takes place through the autonomic nervous system and the HPA axis with its stress hormones cortisol, norepinephrine, etc. The brain can also produce symptoms spontaneously, for example if the sensory apparatus is understimulated. This is known from e.g. phantom limb pain, and it is shown by PET scanning that tinnitus looks like a hallucination. Some studies suggest that the cerebral changes are reversible, including that they are normalised after treatment [128].

PET scan of patients with functional disorders and normal controls during pain stimulation. An increase in activity is seen in the areas corresponding to the pain matrix in figure 6.2, but a smaller increase is seen in the patients than normally. Patients: Contralateral SII, Contralateral thalamus, Contralateral insula. Controls:

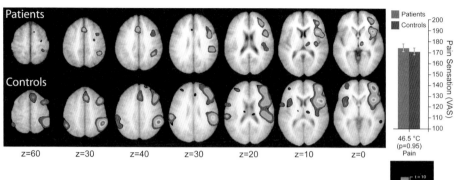

Figure 6.3 Sensation of pain [98]

Conclusion

There seems to be little doubt that biological factors and the CNS are involved in functional disorders, but we know very little about how this happens. As far as the patients are concerned, it is necessary to use a simple explanatory model like the filter theory, hypersensibility or increased symptom production.

Summary

+ A certain hereditary predisposition for functional disorders has been documented.
+ The body responds physiologically to physical or mental stress with arousal, leading to the production of symptoms characteristic of functional disorders.
+ Neurophysiological studies suggest a lack of filter function to irrelevant bodily stimuli in patients with functional disorders.
+ In research contexts, PET and f-MRI scans of patients with functional disorders have shown changes compared with healthy controls.

CHAPTER 7

The interaction between the doctor and patients with functional disorders

PER FINK, MARIANNE ROSENDAL, TOMAS TOFT AND ANDREAS SCHRÖDER

Mismatch

A frequent cause of problems in the interaction between the doctor and patient is that a mismatch exists between what the patient wants to achieve or get from the doctor, and what the doctor gives. Prejudices about the patient population are numerous, and obsolete knowledge continues to dominate the perception and treatment of patients with functional disorders. For example, it is a widespread belief among doctors that patients want tests and physical treatment, and that they are reluctant to talk about psychosocial issues. New research suggests, however, that in some cases, it is the doctor who somatises, not the patient, i.e. the doctor wants to focus on physical disease. This is one of the reasons why patients may feel misunderstood. In addition, the doctor's lack of knowledge about functional disorders may contribute to the patient's feeling of not being understood. Table 7.1 summarises some of the misunderstandings that may arise between the doctor and the patient on the basis of their different expectations [130].

Although patients often have considered various explanations for their symptoms (see also Chapter 8), they naturally expect that the doctor can diagnose or exclude a possible physical disease. They thus also expect to be examined by means of commonly used procedures. In primary care, this may for example be a focused physical examination and possible paraclinical tests that can be performed on site and produce an immediate result. The challenge is for the doctor to balance between; on the one hand, investigating enough to achieve both a mental effect in the patient and to even feel that he/she is navigating safe diagnostic waters and, on the other hand, not undertaking more tests than necessary and proportionate to warrant the absence of a suspected physical disease.

Table 7.1. Mismatch between the patient's expectations and what the doctor offers

What the patient wants	What the patient gets
To know the cause	No diagnosis
Explanations and information	Poor explanations that have nothing to do with their needs or worries
Advice and treatment	Inadequate advice
Reassurance	No reassurance
To be taken seriously by an empathic and competent doctor	A feeling that the doctor is uninterested or thinks that the symptoms are trivial
Emotional support	No emotional support

The doctor's contribution (iatrogenic factors)

The way in which the treatment system and the doctors react to and manage patients with functional symptoms can be instrumental in causing the patients to become ill and to maintain the patients in a sick role with subsequent chronification as a result. The pathological circle of tests and attempts at intervention that may be seen in patients with functional disorders is powerfully illustrated by Sternbach [298] and Quill [131] and reproduced in Figure 7.1. The figure also illustrates the close, almost symbiotic interactions that can be between a doctor and a patient with a functional disorder.

One may often wonder how it is possible that patients with functional disorders have been through such a large number of futile investigations and treatment attempts and so much hospitalisation and surgery. Why

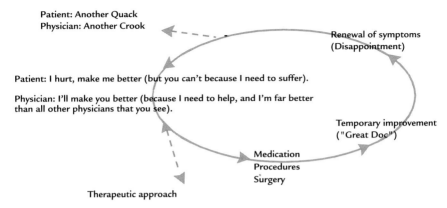

Figure 7.1 The vicious circle in doctor-patient contact. Modified after Sternbach and Quill [298;131]

do doctors continue to investigate and "treat" despite the fact that there is no organic basis for the symptoms? Why is it not possible to say 'stop'? Part of the rationale for this seemingly irrational reaction among doctors is described below.

The fear of overlooking a physical disease

Fear of overlooking a physical disease is the cause frequently quoted by general practitioners as their reason for conducting investigations for which medical indications are rarely found. Recent studies of how often an organic basis for functional symptoms is overlooked, however, show that this rarely happens, especially where disease trajectories are long; actually in only the 3-4% of cases [17;132-134]. And it is probably even rarer that organic disease is overlooked in patients with functional disorders than in patients without such disorders, since the former have a low threshold for consulting their general practitioner [135].

Most doctors will probably agree that it is impossible to completely avoid overlooking physical diseases or making a wrong diagnosis, no matter how careful you are. Fortunately, serious consequences for the patient are probably only seen in very few cases because the diagnosis and hence the treatment are in most cases just delayed.

A frequently quoted argument for carrying out an investigation on a dubious indication is that "one can never be 100% sure". This is true, and it is also the best argument for the need to set a reasonable limit and not continue to carry out investigations. The desire for a utopic, high level of security, is often rooted more in the doctor's need than in the concern for the patient's best interests, for example that the doctor wants to show that he/she has done their duty or because he/she is professionally uncertain. The price for this strategy is paid by the large group of patients with functional disorders, not just in terms of discomfort due to the many unnecessary examinations, but also in terms of their risk of incurring iatrogenic harm. Furthermore, an excessive examination programme may maintain the patient in the sick role and cause chronification and may unduly delay or even prevent sufficient treatment. Functional and mental disorders should be treated with the same seriousness as physical diseases, both in the light of the high mortality in mental disorders and the significant impact it can have on patients' functioning.

It may seem paradoxical that many doctors are likely to continue to look for an explanation of functional disorders, even when they have been diagnosed and the patient has been thoroughly assessed. There are many physical diseases whose underlying cause we do not know, such as essential hypertension. The causes of hypertension may be many; yet, we do not continue to look for the cause, but are satisfied to conclude that it is "essential" when a "reasonable" test battery has been completed.

The fear of complaints and prosecution

The fear of public blame among colleagues or in the press or even the fear of being prosecuted for malpractice can also be a powerful motivation for the numerous investigations [17,136]. In order to guard themselves against subsequent criticism, doctors may feel inclined to carry out tests and take samples that from a medical point of view may seem questionable. In the United States, "defensive" tests and samples are part of daily practice, and one can fear that it is now also becoming the case in Denmark.

Absence of other treatment

Knowledge of more recent psychosocial treatment principles and methods may be limited among non-psychiatric doctors. Some doctors fear that referral to a psychiatrist or another psychosocial treatment option may result in long-term therapy from which patients show little significant improvement. If the doctor does not have confidence in the psychosocial treatment, he may despite the lack of indication opt, instead, to try a biomedical "treatment" while "giving the patient the benefit of the doubt", because "you cannot be sure that the treatment does not work". The consequence of this approach is that patients are not diagnosed and, hence, possibly forego effective treatment.

Unfortunately, the negative, stereotyped attitudes towards the general psychiatric treatment services are not without substance. Many general psychiatrists and psychologists have only a scarce knowledge of functional disorders and their treatment. In addition, in psychiatry there is a tendency to perceive the functional disorders as mild cases of mental disturbances or disorders that do not belong in psychiatry, and which psychiatry does not have the capacity to treat [137;138]. This perception is probably rooted in the fact that the psychiatrist rarely sees these patients, because they, by their very nature, primarily attend non-psychiatric doctors because they are presenting with physical complaints. The result of these positions is that a group of patients, some of whom are very ill, do not receive sufficient treatment, and that the healthcare system continues to allow these patients "to float around the system". There are today only a few specialised treatment clinics.

Lack of understanding of the nature and character of the illness

A few patients with functional disorders can be insistent on further investigations to exclude various physical diseases. Some doctors may think that the patient thereby is just being tested and receives the treatment the patient himself has asked for, and that this is, in other words, the patient's own responsibility [131;136]. This argument rests on the misconception that man's actions are always rational. The desire for more studies or a specific treatment may be rational in the patient's eyes, i.e. given the knowledge the patient has about disease and treatment. We must bear in mind, however, that for many patients, the main source of knowledge about health and disease is newspapers and magazines where the information may be of varying quality. In some cases, the messages carried are simplistic, sensationalist stories about overlooked or mistreated disease or foreign miraculous cures. Furthermore, wishful thinking is a natural mental reaction in a difficult situation. The patient should therefore not be given the entire responsibility for his or her treatment and diagnostic assessment, and the patient is not always acting in his or her own best interests, because he/she does not have the prerequisites to make the right decisions, and because he or she is, of course, emotionally highly committed to his or her own illness. The doctor must therefore maintain an overview and apply his professional expertise to help the patient make the right decisions, and this is not possible if he reduces himself to a "body mechanic" who does not have as his main concern the patient's best interest and well-being from an overall perspective.

You may see doctors conduct non-routine examinations just to convince patients that they are mistaken in their assumption that they suffer from a certain disease. This may sometimes seem reassuring, but not to mentally unstable patients or patients with a functional disorder [139]. Rather, they may interpret it as if "there's probably still something about this" because the doctors took samples (on the implicit understanding that the doctor was also in doubt).

Lack of knowledge in handling functional disorders

Many doctors are trained within a predominantly biomedical disease model and feel uncertain when encountering mental aspects. It may therefore require an extra effort to take a broad bio-psycho-social approach to a problem and to pursue multiple tracks simultaneously; which may even be true for GPs who are trained to do so. In many cases, the doctor will therefore choose to resort to the familiar routine of tests and attempts at treatment. This can happen either by the doctor focusing narrowly on clarifying a physical disease (*searching for a disease*) or on a single, discrete and current problem, which is then examined by the usual routine in which a doctor avoid making a more comprehensive assessment of the patient's other problems (*going by the routine*) [140].

The doctor can take refuge in ascribing the patient's complaints to some random discoveries, such as attributing back pain to X-ray findings that may also be seen in asymptomatic individuals. Both the doctor and patient may be satisfied that they have found the "explanation" for the symptoms, but the symptoms almost always return after some time.

Some GPs follow the patient's wishes for examinations and tests on the grounds that the patient would otherwise see another doctor. A change of GP would lead to further examinations, samples, admittances and treatment attempts until the new GP gets to know the patient (see also Figure 7.1). The history may repeat itself. To protect the patient from unnecessary suffering, the GP may accept the patient's wish for more tests. It should be noted that such a strategy *may* be appropriate if it is conducted in a sober and judicious manner and on a sure indication and hence prevents the patient from suffering additional discomfort and the risk of iatrogenic harm.

The doctor's personality and perception of his/her role as a medical professional

Most mental problems are common to man. All people have various "raw nerves", i.e. things they are sensitive about and have difficulty handling. Conversations about mental and social problems can therefore become unpleasant because they can provide reminders or remind the doctor about his or her own problems [141]. Some doctors are trying to solve this problem by avoiding having "subjective" contact with the patient and instead maintaining an "objective" view of the symptoms the patient presents.

Some doctors believe that their task is merely to investigate and deal with physical problems and that, in all cases, you should first rule out a physical disease as the cause of the problem. They feel that they are themselves not equipped to explore psychosocial problems and may think that this type of problems has nothing to do with physical problems [131,136].

Doctors have often gone into the profession with an idealistic attitude: Doctors must be good, kind, knowing, self-sacrificing and helpful. A doctor has an inherent urge to prove to himself and to others that he/she is competent and meets these qualities mentioned [141]. The patient may put heavy pressure on the doctor by appealing to the emotional part of the doctor's self-image with statements like: "I will do everything to get well"; "I cannot handle it anymore, you must help"; "It is you who are the doctor". The doctor who is not familiar with psychosocial treatment will be particularly inclined in a situation where pressure is felt to resort to the biomedical model with which he/she is most familiar [142-145].

Modesty

Some doctors feel that they violate the patient's shyness by asking questions about emotional well-being, just like a gynaecological or rectal examination may be felt as intimidating [136;141]. You sometimes get the impression that doctors may find it easier to perform these examinations than asking the patient how he or she feels about oneself. Whether a patient feels intimidated or not depends on whether he or she understands why the topic is being raised or a certain examination performed.

Pandora's Box or the fear of loss of control

Many doctors have found that once they begin to ask about the patient's problems, the patient shows a large, pent-up need to talk about these problems and to get emotional support. It may seem completely overwhelming to the doctor who does not know how he/she may stop the patient again in a compassionate way, let alone how he/she can help the patient with these apparently massive problems [146].

The doctor may also be afraid of the patient's reaction (if the patient leaves, gets angry, cries, etc.) and by performing an additional test "just in case", this confrontation may be avoided.

The fear of dependency

The GP may choose not to raise psycho-social issues because he is afraid that the patient will become dependent on him and that this dependency cannot cease again [136,141]. If the GP is aware of both his own and the patient's limits, and talks directly with the patient about these limits, this should, however, not be a problem. If the framework for raising these issues is discussed with the patient in a sensitive way, the patient will rarely take offence. On the contrary, most patients will find it reassuring that the conversation unfolds within a set framework, and that the GP sets this framework. In those cases where it is a problem, it may be a good idea to discuss the matter with a colleague or a psychiatrist.

Time pressure

The GP may think that there is no time to take a more comprehensive approach to the patient's problem by obtaining a psychosocial medical history and to take care of mental disorders. This may, however, be quickly accomplished if time is used effectively and in a structured manner when taking a medical history. It also appears that a sufficiently thorough investigation and explanation given to the patient at the first contact will save much time over a period, because the patient will not return due to the uncertainty that arises if questions are left unanswered.

Moreover, it has been documented that time may be saved by asking the patient directly about mental problems and social issues, because you may hence avoid so-called "door handle" questions where the patient, leaving the surgery with his hand on the door handle, raises a seemingly casual question: "By the way …". [147].

Summary

Iatrogenic factors in functional disorders
+ A frequent cause of problems in the interaction between doctors and patient is that there often is a mismatch between what the patient wants to achieve or get from the doctor and what the doctor gives.
+ The ways in which the healthcare system works and doctors respond to and manage patients with functional symptoms may contribute to the patient's illness, maintain the patient in the sick role and cause chronification.
  - The doctor's fear of overlooking a physical disease, get a complaint or be prosecuted.
  - Absence of other treatments.
  - Lack of skills in dealing with functional disorders or lack of understanding of the disorder.
  - The doctor's own modesty, personality, perception of the medical profession, or fear of loss of control.
  - Time pressure and fear of patient dependency.

CHAPTER 8

The patient's symptom perception and illness beliefs

PER FINK, MARIANNE ROSENDAL, TOMAS TOFT AND ANDREAS SCHRÖDER.

People respond differently to symptoms in terms of when treatment is sought, which symptoms constitute a reason for encounter, self-treatment, etc. It is primarily our own interpretations and beliefs that determine whether we perceive something as a normal bodily sensation or as a sign of a disease/symptom for which we seek medical help or treatment. In other words, we have different illness behaviours. Illness behaviour can be divided into:

- *Treatment-seeking behaviour*, i.e. our behaviour in relation to treatment and healthcare in general.
- *Social illness behaviour*, i.e. our behaviour in relation to family, friends, work and society in general.
- *Self-care and self-treatment*, i.e. our lifestyle, ways of life and attempts to treat ourselves.

Illness behaviour is determined by the way we interpret, evaluate and perceive symptoms, i.e. our *illness perception* [148]. Thus, cognitive and emotional factors that motivate a given behaviour, and illness behaviour are therefore shaped by cultural, social and other learned practices, including upbringing. Illness perception and illness behaviour are crucial determinants of our healthcare use, but illness perception and illness behaviour only partially correlate with the severity and nature of physical diseases as judged from biomedical parameters [149].

Health psychology distinguishes between at least five main dimensions of the patient's illness perception [150]. These are listed in Table 8.1.

Table 8.1 Dimensions of illness perception

The 5 main dimensions in the patient's understanding of his own illness:
• *Identity:* The designation the patient uses (e.g. tension headache) and the symptoms that the patient attributes to illness.
• *Cause:* Does the patient, for example, think that the illness is solely due to a physical disease that psychosocial factors have played a role in, or that other causes are at play?
• *Duration:* Does the patient think that the illness is short-lived or does he/she fear chronic illness?
• *Consequences:* Does the patient, for example, think that he/she will return to work, will be much troubled, be sick-listed etc.?
• *Treatment and control:* Does the patient think that he/she will be well again, that treatment will help, and that he/she will be able, to a greater or lesser extent, to influence his symptoms, or does the patient feel entirely helpless and without any influence on his symptoms or illness?

The patient's own symptom perception and illness beliefs are important for his or her morbidity and functional impairment, not only within the context of functional and mental disorders, but also in well-defined physical diseases, where one's own perception may be crucial for the prognosis in terms of subjective well-being, functioning, compliance and use of health care services.

Figure 8.1 shows a basic model for how people perceive and evaluate physical sensations and symptoms. The model takes as its premise that all people daily experience non-pathological physical sensations or symptoms that both the patient and the doctor might misinterpret as signs of a physical disease [17]. Sensations or symptoms may stem from natural physiological processes or disease. This process is universal to all people, and it is of a continuous nature. The process ranges from the totally unconscious to the all-pervasive, for example a patient with health anxiety will think of nothing but his/her possible illness, or the patient with a serious bodily disease will think about it all the time.

The process can have a tonus or excitability that varies from person to person depending on the biological conditions and acquired experiences.

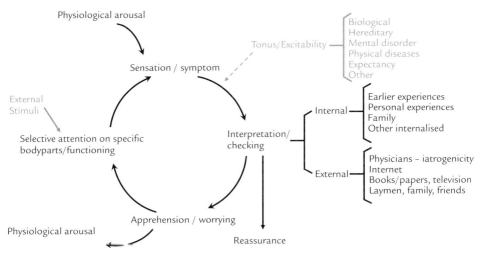

Figure 8.1 Illness perception and illness beliefs [17]

For example, a person who has been cured of cancer will be sensitive to the symptoms he or she previously had in connection with the cancer. The general level of excitability is also influenced by moods and mental stress. A person who is depressed or suffers from anxiety will be more sensitive and concerned and thus have a lower threshold for detecting symptoms. Expectations also have a bearing on the tonus of the process [151].

Previous experience and internal evaluation

All humans have a relatively stable *sensation or symptom panorama* with which they are confident. This confidentiality builds up through life in a continuous process. When girls enter puberty, for example, they become familiar with new symptoms in connection with their period, and these experiences are added to their symptom panorama. Patients also enter new symptoms of chronic disease into their panorama, and the patient begins to consider whether there may be another cause, or whether the disease has worsened only when changes in intensity, type or composition of symptoms appear. Experience with symptoms from various diseases will also become part of a person's internalised frame of reference. For example, most have had the flu and have learned that it is associated with pain behind the eyes, headache, fever, upper respiratory tract symptoms, etc. If a person gets these symptoms, he or she will often think that it is probably the flu, and will not be worried or seek medical help. The sensation panorama is influenced by cultural and social factors, whereas the severity of a symptom means less to our interpretation of whether it may be a sign of illness or not. Even the strongest physical sensations may be completely normal, e.g. heavy dyspnoea and palpitations after running, and will therefore not be interpreted by the individual as a sign of illness. This may be illustrated from the illness behaviour of a family that for generations has been suffering from severe migraine, resulting in hemiplegia [152]. Members of the family have rarely sought medical help because their symptoms were well-known and even self-limiting, and so far no doctor has been able to help.

External sources

When the internal evaluation of the sensations/symptoms is insufficient, individuals seek information or help from *external sources*. These sources could be family members, colleagues, books, the Internet or magazines, etc. Finally, the patient can consult a GP for reassurance or treatment. The GP's information and reaction will be of great importance, as the response and any questions asked could strengthen or weaken the patient's interest in special symptoms/organs. These experiences can then be internalised into the patient's experience.

Information from various external sources may cause a person to change perception of well-known sensations so that they are suddenly misinterpreted as signs of illness. Medical students may have experienced this on their own bodies when reading pathology. The external information initiates the process outlined in Figure 8.1. The concern to which the new information gives rise will cause the mind to focus attention on the body part that harbours the suspected disorder and from where the symptoms are expected to originate. We all know this phenomenon: you're having a headache and begin to test if there should also be other symptoms. This causes new sensations/symptoms to come to your mind, e.g. that you feel tired or uninspired, and these new symptoms will also be interpreted both in relation to the person's own experience and external sources. The result is that the person is either reassured or becomes more nervous that the symptoms can be signs of illness. The process may be self-perpetuating because the patient may wrongly attribute the physical symptoms that accompany nervousness or anxiety to the disease. When the process is initiated by external influences, it is also called *suggestion* and *autosuggestion*. The epidemic of allergic reactions to copy paper [153], which received much publicity in 1979, serves as an example of the *(auto) suggestive element*. Investigation of this phenomenon revealed that allergic reactions were caused by only one particular kind of copy paper. Most of those who complained of allergic reactions had never been in contact with this type of copy paper. After the study was published and the copy paper in question was withdrawn from the market, the number of cases swiftly fell to zero. Medical literature and press often feature such new epidemics. Recent examples would be the chronic whiplash and multiple chemical sensitivity, electricity and radiation from various electronic instruments.

Summary

+ All humans daily experience spontaneous bodily sensations, but how these sensations are perceived and interpreted varies.
+ Symptom perception depends, among others, on the nervous system's current perception tonus, which is influenced, among others, by genetic factors, the patient's current emotional state and the patient's expectations. Attention to a symptom can reinforce its perception.
+ Internal evaluation of the symptoms is the patient's primary understanding of the condition formed on the basis of learning in childhood and previous experience.
+ External evaluation most often takes place when the internal evaluation does not suffice. Information may be obtained from family members, the internet, books, magazines, encyclopaedias, etc. The doctor is usually regarded as one among many experts by the patients.
+ Symptom interpretation spans a continuum depending on upbringing, family myths, previous experiences, state of mind, and how the disorder is handled within the healthcare system.
+ The patient's own understanding of the disease and morbidity shapes the course and prognosis, among others in the light of the patient's hypothesis about the consequences and his or her sense of personal control over the disease.
+ Illness behaviour has a larger impact on health care use than symptom severity. Illness behaviour is primarily driven by the patient's symptom perception and illness beliefs.

PART II

TREATMENT

CHAPTER 9

Overview of treatment options

PER FINK, MARIANNE ROSENDAL AND ANDREAS SCHRÖDER

The results of treatment of functional disorders seem to be quite good. A number of meta-analyses are unanimously showing a positive effect of psychological treatment of functional somatic syndromes such as chronic fatigue syndrome, fibromyalgia, non-cardiogenic chest pain and irritable bowel syndrome (Table 9.1). A number of meta-analyses are unanimous in showing a positive effect of psychological treatment on functional syndromes such as chronic fatigue syndrome, fibromyalgia, non-cardiogenic chest pain and irritable bowel syndrome (Table 9.1). This applies notably to cognitive behavioural therapies [24;25]. Psychodynamic and psycho-pharmacological treatments have also shown positive results. Systematic reviews examining the effect across syndrome diagnoses come to the same result [23; 26; 58; 154-156].

In a recent Danish randomised controlled trial, patients with chronic multi-organ system *bodily distress syndrome* received cognitive behavioural therapy in groups following a thorough assessment at a specialised treatment centre (a detailed description of the treatment is given below). One of the results was that the same approach may be applied in patients with functional disorders regardless of which symptom is most prominent, or which syndrome diagnosis(es) the patients may previously have been given [23;58].

Patients with functional disorders are burdened by somatic symptoms and primarily experience that they are suffering from a physical condition.

Table 9.1. Evidence for antidepressants, exercise and psychological interventions in different subtypes of bodily distress. (Symptom profiles are ordered according to the BDS concept; whereas references refer to the mentioned diagnostic categories. Evidence ratings are based on reference 26 and recent meta-analyses or high-quality randomised controlled trials. Only the most important references are listed).

Symptom profile (BDS subtype) and corresponding functional somatic syndrome or diagnostic label / Type of treatment	GS-type Chronic Fatigue Syndrome	MS-type Fibromyalgia	GI-type Irritable Bowel Syndrome	CP-type Non-cardiac chest pain	Multi-organ type Multiple Medically Unexplained Symptoms and somatisation disorder
Antidepressants	+ [26;157]	+++ [158]	+++ [159;160]	?	++ [156;161;162]
Exercise	+++ [157;163;164]	+++ [165;166]	?	?	+ [167]
Psychological treatment (mainly CBT)	+++ [157;168;169]	+++ [170;171]	++ [159;172;173]	++ [174]	+++ [156;161;162;167] [25;58;175;176]

+++ strong evidence
++ moderate evidence
+ weak evidence
? no evidence, or lack of studies

They therefore, naturally, mainly contact non-psychiatric doctors. Today, most treatment thus takes place in primary care and to a limited extent in general hospital units and outpatient clinics. Moreover, many psychiatrists and psychologists are not familiar with the treatment of these disorders and may find it difficult to handle new somatic symptom complaints during therapy. The treatment of functional disorders is therefore not only a psychiatric issue.

The treatment of functional disorders should be based on a *stepped care* approach in which we must try to define who is responsible for what and at which level of specialisation the patient is best treated (illustrated in Figure

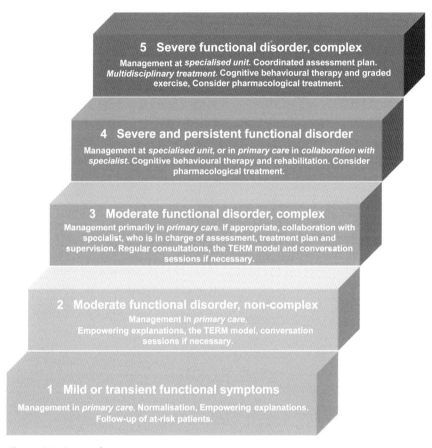

Figure 9.1 Stepped care

9.1). This decision should include considerations of practicability based, among others, on an assessment of available resources, what is acceptable to the patient, an assessment of the severity of the disorder and the doctor's own competence within the area.

The specialist's resources are brought to their best use in a *shared care* model in which the specialist provides support and serves as a consultant to primary care and the specialised general hospital section and only has direct patient contact in difficult cases. Unfortunately, there are currently no such systematic offers of *shared care* for patients with functional disorders in most countries including Denmark.

The principle behind *stepped care* is that the recommended treatment depends on where the patient is on the severity spectrum ranging from mild cases with functional symptoms to severe and complex cases of functional somatic syndromes or multi-organ *bodily distress syndrome*.

The medical specialist and general hospital specialist departments

Table 9.2 outlines the role of a general hospital specialist unit. To avoid that the patient embarks on an odyssey through the treatment system, it is important that the specialist is very clear in his/her communication with the patient and the referring doctor to avoid further, unnecessary investigations and treatment attempts. This also affords the patient and the general practitioner with the best possibilities for continuing their pursuit of other, more relevant treatment options. Referring to a specialist assessment, the general practitioner can speak with more confidence and authority. There should generally be a medical indication for any investigation, and no investigations should be conducted based solely on patient requests or to reassure the patient that nothing is wrong. Several studies have shown that investigations per se do not alter the patient's beliefs or eliminate his or her concern, but may, instead, help maintain or intensify worrying. In some cases, an investigation might be required to reassure the doctor and hence prevent new referrals and investigations.

The medical specialist should have essential knowledge of functional disorders and bodily distress, so that they are capable of establishing this differential diagnosis or at least keeping it in mind as a possibility. There is a significant risk that a wrong diagnosis is pursued if the doctor focuses only on symptoms that are relevant to his or her own specialty and the disease that he or she suspects.

As discussed in Chapter 7, there is often a mismatch between the patient's expectations to the consultation and the answers they actually get. The doctor should try to identify the patient's expectations and to anticipate questions in order to be able to answer these in the best way and later to counter any unrealistic expectations.

Table 9.2 The role of the specialist centre/the specialist in the treatment of patients with functional disorders.

+ Rule out, within reason, the possibility of physical disease or any injury that may be treated.
+ Tell the patient in an empathic manner that there are no signs of organic disease within the area of your expertise.
+ Explain to the patient that there is no medical indication for any further medical investigations or tests within your area of expertise.
+ Be honest, show respect and be professional.
+ Make the diagnosis of functional disorder (or similar terms, e.g. *Bodily distress syndrome*).
+ Avoid contributing to placing the patient in a sick role.
+ Attempt to address the patient's questions and expectations, both the clear and the unspoken ones.
+ Coordinate treatment with the patient's GP and other doctors with whom the patient is in contact. Feed back in a clear and unequivocal way to other healthcare professionals.
+ Consider referral to psychiatric assessment or specialist units for functional disorders.
+ See also treatment methods Chapters 10-13.

The general practitioner (GP)

In most cases, the GP is the health care professional who is in the best position to treat mild and moderate cases, especially in countries with a family doctor system. Depending on the GP's qualifications and capabilities, severe or chronic cases could be treated in primary care even if such cases should ideally be managed in a shared care model where a specialist helps the GP with supervision and possibly with direct patient contact.

Specialised treatment

Specialised treatment for this patient group is extremely scarce world-wide, perhaps with the exception of Germany. In Denmark, The Research Clinic for Functional Disorders and Psychosomatics was established in 1999 at Aarhus University Hospital. This is, to the best of the authors' belief, the first clinic in the world specialised in functional disorders only. Since 2004, a treatment programme that combines graded exercise therapy with methods from cognitive behavioural therapy has been developed at the department. The treatment, which has been designated STreSS (*specialised treatment*

Specialised Treatment for Severe Bodily Distress Syndromes (STreSS)

Module	Week	Content and Objectives
1st Module	1	**Introduction to STreSS** Objectives: Enhancing motivation to deal with painful and disabling bodily symptoms. Full acknowledgement of patients' suffering. Introduction to cognitive behavioural therapy. Introduction of group members.
2nd Module	2	**Bodily symptoms and their interpretation** Objectives: Registration and differentiation of bodily symptoms. Challenging inflexible symptom attributions.
3rd Module	3	**Illness perceptions. Stress response. Treatment goals.** Objectives: Diagnostic labels for and subtypes of bodily distress syndromes. Biological, psychological and social factors contributing to the development and maintenance of bodily distress. Impact of negative illness perceptions. Defining individual treatment goals for each patient.
4th Module	4	**Negative automatic thoughts and dysfunctional behaviours** Objectives: (Re-)Connecting bodily symptoms with emotions, thoughts and behaviours. For each patient, identification of perpetuating factors (thoughts and behaviours) that contribute to disability.
5th Module	6	**Cognitive distortions and emotional awareness** Objectives: Ongoing work with the connection of bodily symptoms, emotions, thoughts and behaviours. Identification of cognitive distortions. Construction of alternative responses. Enhancing emotional awareness.
6th Module	8	**From illness behaviour to health behaviour I** Objectives: Ongoing work with the connection of bodily symptoms, emotions, thoughts and behaviours. Looking back: connecting life events and bodily distress. Looking forward: boosting pleasurable activities.
7th Module	10	**From illness behaviour to health behaviour II** Objectives: Restoring sleep, balanced diet, and physical exercise. Evaluating social network and interpersonal relationships. Evaluating work status. Revision and adjustment of individual treatment goals.
8th Module	12	**Becoming your own therapist. Relapse prevention** Objectives: Adaption of life-style to improved functioning. Recapitulation of dysfunctional thoughts and behaviours, and construction of alternative beliefs. Providing problem solving skills. Drawing up individual treatment manual for possible relapse.
9th Module	16	**How to maintain learned skills and coping strategies** Objectives: Review of concepts taught and skills learned in the STreSS programme. Definition of individual goals for the next 3 months. Recapitulation and farewell.

Each module consists of 3.5 hours. Treatment is delivered by 2 therapists in groups of 9 patients . Each patient is allocated a contact therapist who is primarily responsible for his or her treatment. The treatment manual is available at www.functionaldisorders.dk

Figure 9.2 Overview of a cognitive-based treatment programme at a specialist centre

for severe *Bodily distress syndrome*), is organised as group therapy and can be administered to patients with functional syndromes and somatoform disorders (Figure 9.2). STreSS has been shown to outperform the current "standard treatment" and to have a moderate effect on patients' self-reported physical health and a *number needed to treat* of 5 for therapeutic response (defined as an improvement of at least half a standard deviation on the primary outcome measure). When asked directly, 60% indicated that the treatment received had significantly improved their situation [58]. Treatment of this group of patients is currently undertaken by psychiatrists with a special expertise in functional disorders. It has so far not been established if parts of the treatment may in the future be delegated to other health care professionals such as nurses or psychologists with special training. Severe or complicated cases of health anxiety may also be managed in specialised clinics, but the current capacity to undertake such treatment is also very limited world-wide.

Pharmacological treatment

A concomitant anxiety disorder, depression or other psychiatric disorder in patients with functional disorders can be effectively treated according to current guidelines. Antidepressants (SSRIs, NaSSAs, TCAs, SNRIs) may be effective in both health anxiety and other functional disorders, even in patients who are not depressed [24;161;177-180]. Treatment with psychoactive medication is occasionally hampered by patients' reluctance to take medication. However, such opposition is often rooted in the patient's belief that the doctor prescribes psychoactive medication because he thinks that the patient is depressed.

In functional disorders, psychopharmacological treatment is targeted against disturbances of symptom perception and the central inhibition of pain and not against a suspected underlying depression. A thorough explanation of the indication, offering perhaps examples from the use of antidepressants in pain treatment, can often clear these misunderstandings and improve compliance.

Furthermore, antiepileptics (gabapentin, pregabalin, lamotrigin, carbamazepin) used in pain management presumably also have an effect [180] except in health anxiety where these have not been tested. Any treatment should take into account that patients with functional disorders are often more sensitive to side effects, and treatment should start at a lower dose than normal (*start low-go slow*). Furthermore, only drugs that can be monitored in serum should be used in order to allow evaluation of side effects and compliance. In some cases, specific symptom treatment may be indicated, e.g. motility modifying drugs for irritable bowel syndrome [179].

Summary

Treatment options

+ Treatment should follow a *stepped care* principle.
+ Patients are burdened by physical symptoms, and treatment of functional disorders is therefore not only a psychiatric issue.
+ Specialist doctors in relevant specialties should be familiar with functional disorders to avoid misdiagnosis and maltreatment within their own specialty.
+ General practitioners should be able to treat mild and moderate cases of functional disorders and could be included in shared care regimes with specialist centres for treatment of severe and chronic cases.
+ There is evidence of effect of a specific treatment programme conducted by specialists, e.g. in the form of cognitive behavioural therapy.
+ Some patients with severe disorders could benefit from medical treatment in the form of antidepressants or anti-epileptics.
+ Patients with functional disorders are often more sensitive to side effects. It is recommended to start with a lower dose and to step up medication slower than usual (*start low – go slow*).

CHAPTER 10

Ensuring a good doctor-patient relationship

PER FINK, MARIANNE ROSENDAL AND ANDREAS SCHRÖDER

A good doctor-patient relationship rests on mutual respect and trust, but in patients with functional disorders, it is also a prerequisite that the treatment is structured with clear agreements, clean lines, openness, and that the doctor is clear about the diagnosis. It is necessary that the doctor knows and understands the nature of functional disorders in order not to be continually unsure about the diagnosis. The doctor must be conscious of his or her role in the diagnosis and the treatment (see Chapter 9).

Doctors who are managing patients with severe functional disorders may sometimes experience a feeling of professional insufficiency and thus feel that patient contact is stressful. In some cases, these patients would be better treated in specialised health care in collaboration with primary care, but this is rarely possible in the present health care system. If the advice on the management of these disorders, as specified in Chapter 11, is followed, both the doctor and the patient may avoid much frustration. The following section discusses some of the specific characteristics that are important to have in mind to maintain a good doctor-patient relationship, even when it comes to patients with severe functional disorders.

Avoid assuming a responsibility that is not yours

The relationship between the doctor and patients with functional disorders most often goes wrong because the doctor willingly, or because of the patient's pressure, assumes a responsibility which he/she is unable to live up to. It is natural that the patient desires that the doctor removes the symptoms and therefore may wish an intervention focused on a particular organ, but this causes problems if the symptoms are not caused by any pathological changes. In a British study at a gynaecological ward, consultations due to abdominal disorders without organic basis were analysed, and consultations that led to hysterectomy were compared with those that did not lead to hysterectomy [142]. The patients typically focused on their subjective symptoms and the consequences for their lives and the quality of their lives. They could sometimes be insistent in their demands that the gynaecologist do something here and now. The patient, for example, put pressure on the doctor by referring to previously failed treatment attempts and by devaluing previously met therapists and previous treatments – the implication being: "If you do not help me, you're just as bad", "Nothing has helped me, somebody has do something!". In the consultations that led to hysterectomy despite the lack of an organic basis, the gynaecologist typically accepted that the consultation was conducted on the patient's terms. The topic was the subjective effects and symptoms caused by the disorder. These are areas where the patient is the absolute expert.

Inversely, in consultations that did not lead to hysterectomy, the gynaecologist took a firm position, saying that he had "seen inside the patient" and that he had seen with his own eyes that nothing was wrong and therefore would not operate. The doctor stood firm within his area of competence, i.e. organic change and physical disease, and argued that he had performed due investigations and found no sign of body changes.

It should be remembered that in the above examples, the doctor's primary responsibility is to investigate and treat physical disease and not to remove abdominal symptoms, which may be rooted in other causes, including functional disorders. The doctor can only help the patient by providing guidance based on factual arguments. It is of no help to remove the uterus if the patient has abdominal symptoms and there is no organ pathology – the doctor must be firm in this regard. The patient cannot challenge the doctor's area of expertise and expert decision that there is "nothing organic to treat". One should thus not accept that the patient makes the doctor responsible for a *physical* therapy, but rather offer to help the patient to explore other options when a biomedical approach is not appropriate. In this context, it is important to accept and express understanding that the patient may have troublesome abdominal symptoms, although nothing is wrong with her uterus.

Form of communication

Patients with severe functional disorders often use a form of communication that, naturally, focuses on their subjective history of suffering and its consequences. The patient's *psycho-social form of communication* may cause the two parties to talk past each other – the doctor is talking about biomedical *facts*, and the patient about symptoms and suffering; in which case the patient will feel misunderstood or the conversation will take place on the terms of only one of the parties. If the patient sets the agenda alone, communication will often be entirely emotional and action-oriented ("I feel bad, do something!"). Recognition of the symptoms, empathic responses to patients' emotional statements, but maintaining diagnostic and therapeutic principles can help build bridges in communication. If the patient tries to make the doctor responsible for his or her problems by maintaining that it is only a physical problem, which the doctor should be able to handle, it is important that the doctor maintains that within his or her area of expertise in physical diseases, there are no organic explanations and appropriate biomedical treatment options. It is important to insist that the problem is best tackled by adopting a broader approach, including involvement of the psychosocial aspects. This is consistent with the approach in chronic illnesses that cannot be cured, e.g. in a patient who is disabled by paresis following a stroke. In this case, the biomedical treatment options are extremely limited, but rehabilitation and psychosocial interventions are crucial to success.

Acceptance of the limits of medicine

Patients with functional disorders consult a doctor, among other reasons, because they expect that medicine has a cure for their problem. The patient may believe that he or she is suffering from an unrecognised physical disease since "the doctors cannot figure out what is wrong with me". It is important in an early phase to uncover the patient's illness understanding and any myths and misconceptions and in an empathetic way tell the patient what is suggested by medical evidence and what are currently the most effective treatments for functional disorders.

A physiological explanation for the patient's symptoms is often beneficial. It is also important to outline the medical limits of treatment, including talking with the patient about the thoughts he / she may have had about potential biomedical treatment. Cognitive therapies and pharmacotherapy often only have moderate effect in chronic functional disorders. This may indicate that medical science has not yet developed interventions that can fully restore the body's symptom perception; or that lasting biological changes in the brain's way of processing and experiencing bodily sensations occur; and that these changes cannot be influenced by medical and psychotherapeutic intervention. On the other hand, some patients become completely asymptomatic, and we must therefore continue to send the message that the patient may become better.

If you have asked the patient about his or her expectations during the consultation, it will be easier to prioritise time and avoid stress due to a full waiting room. If the patient's illness beliefs and opposition to anything other than biomedical explanations suggest that it may be difficult to reach a common understanding, a new appointment allowing ample time for preparation should be scheduled. Time pressure all too often makes it tempting to do nothing. This solution will usually prove time-consuming, because the untreated patient will often return again and again with continued symptoms and renewed concerns.

Summary

Advice on how to build a good relationship with a patient with a functional disorder

+ Be sure what the diagnosis is.
+ Be conscious of your role in the treatment.
+ Ensure structure and clear agreements on consultation and treatment to prevent uncertainty.
+ Do not assume a responsibility that is not yours.
+ Do not let the conversation take place exclusively at a psychosocial communication level: The patient who has a functional disorder can communicate distress and expectations for the doctor to act. Doctors should be empathetic, but also firm on medical indications for intervention or non-intervention.
+ Establish together with the patient realistic expectations to the opportunities and limits of medical science.

CHAPTER 11

Primary assessment and treatment (TERM model)

PER FINK, MARIANNE ROSENDAL AND ANDREAS SCHRÖDER

Definition of own task in treatment and assessment

General practitioners encounter many patients with functional symptoms or mild functional disorders. In these cases, using the model below could be instrumental in achieving treatment of the patient during one or a few consultations, probably preventing the development of illness worry and more chronic disorders. In other cases, patients with functional disorders can be highly complex, both *administratively*, for example because they are simultaneously consulting multiple healthcare professionals; *illnes-wise* because they can present a diffuse, non-specific and uncharacteristic clinical picture. Furthermore, they can also be *socially* complex because of sickness absence, rehabilitation, insurance matters, etc. It is therefore important that the doctor is conscious of the task he/she is facing while managing the complex patient (see Figure 9.1 and Table 9.1). It is usually obvious to the general practitioner (GP) that he or she has the responsibility of being a coordinator. At times, the therapeutic responsibility may be fully or partially transferred to another healthcare professional, like a psychiatrist or a specialist clinic. The scope of the general practitioner's responsibility is determined partly by his qualifications and skills, partly by the availability of other treatment options in the district.

Considerations before the consultation

Knowing his patients, the GP, in some cases, may in advance feel that a patient consults him because of functional symptoms. It may be advantageous to try to sharpen one's focus and clarify the basis of such a feeling in advance. A functional disorder should be considered if the patient has previously presented a vague or complicated symptom picture or has not responded as expected to treatment, if there is a repetitive pattern or in other cases where "something is not quite right".

Table 11.1 Consider the following questions before the consultation

- Similar previous reactions
  - is there a pattern of repetitions?
- Signs of or information about previous mental disturbance or disorder?
- Does the patient have a low consultation threshold?
- Is the disorder chronic?
  - if yes, consider scheduling a status consultation.

Patients with functional disorders can present with pronounced subjective suffering and many problems. This may place the GP under considerable pressure to do something immediately, and the consultation may focus on management of only the most urgent problems. It can be frustrating to constantly be "one step behind" and to feel manipulated by the patient's severe and urgent symptoms, rather than being able to take a medical approach to diagnosis and treatment. This can be avoided by the GP being aware of his role and possible treatments. The specialist doctor may be very competent in areas where treatment has documented effect, but should not assume the responsibility for helping patients in areas where there is no documentation, or that do not lie within the doctor's competences. The GP can maintain an overview by preparing himself for the consultation with a patient with a possible functional disorder. Consideration should be given to the elements listed in Table 11.1. Such preparation allows the GP to prepare an agenda before the consultation and to consider which issues should be focused on. It affords him with an opportunity to be proactive instead of reactive.

General conversation techniques

One of the most important psychological aspects of the treatment programme is that patients feel heard and understood. The experience of being heard is a prerequisite for the patient to be open to a nuanced understanding of his illness. Otherwise, the patient may misunderstand the GP's response and think that the GP may not have understood the severity of the symptoms and the extent to which they make it impossible for the patient to live a normal life; a misunderstanding that will strain the doctor-patient relationship. Knowledge of some general conversation techniques is important to achieve this purpose. These techniques are listed in Table 11.2. It should be emphasised that *the spirit is more important than the technique*. It is more important to be attentive and have good contact with the patient than trying to remember a special technique. One should avoid hiding behind various guidelines, surveys, records, computer screens and the like.

Socratic questioning

The central element of Socratic questioning is curiosity. The task is to try to understand how the patient thinks, feels and perceives things. Listen and ask out of interest with an open mind and do not offer explanations, make corrections or give advice in this part of the encounter. What is interesting in this context is not how things are in reality, but the patient's perception of this. It is much easier and perhaps only possible at a later point in time to correct misunderstandings and misconceptions if you know exactly what they are and if you can go into the patient's mode of thinking. People are generally afraid to reveal their ignorance and say something that they think will sound silly to the expert. Misplaced statements, advice, etc. may make the patient feel that he/she has said something stupid. At worst, the patient may feel ridiculed and feel that he/she has lost face.

Neutrality is important because the patient will soon pull away if the GP's preconceived opinions show through. The GP must fight his/her wish to give advice and explanations, because no matter how well-intended they are, the patient will rarely be able to use them if they diverge much from his/her own thinking. In the 17th century, Blaise Pascal wrote: *"People are generally better persuaded by the reasons which they have themselves discovered, than by those which have come into the mind of others".* Those words still apply.

Table 11.2 Interview technique

+	÷

• Socratic questioning technique
  – Be neutral and genuinely curious
  – Use open questions
  – Use encouragement (facilitating)
  – Keep the focus
• Summarise frequently
• Empathy/emotional feedback
• Roll with resistance (rope-a-dope)
• Support self-help and own control
  – Let the patient suggest his own solutions and support the patient's feeling of being able to do something himself (*empowerment*).
	• Closed questions (questions that can be answered by a yes/no)
	• Advice
	• Premature correction
	• Argumentation and confrontation
	• Attempts at persuasion

Use open questions such as: "How do you think?", "What do you think?", "What goes through your head when you feel like this?" If closed questions are used, i.e. questions that can be answered with a yes/no, the GP alone will control the conversation and thus take responsibility, which may feel as a burden for the GP, especially if you are unsure of what to do or where you are heading. The patient may also feel under pressure if many questions are asked, but most patients describe it as more relaxing and safe to be allowed to use their own words. It gives them greater satisfaction if they are given the opportunity to raise issues felt to be important to them and to express their own interpretation. The patient will feel that the GP is listening and will feel understood. The GP can support the patient by encouraging remarks such as "Aha …", "really", "continue" and "tell me more about that". The idea is not that you should remain passive and let the patient control the entire conversation. Patients rightly expect that GPs make sure to respect the time and obtain the necessary information. If the patient raises too many issues by narrating stories or by giving irrelevant information, the GP may focus the conversation, saying for example: "It's interesting to hear how your trip went, but I would like to hear more about …", or "It sounds like something that is important; I would like to hear more about this later, but can we just go back to … ". This way of parking information in order to keep focus may also be used if the patient presents specific wishes early in the consultation: "You mention a sick note, I would like to speak with you about that before we stop today; but right now, I would like to hear something about …".

The Socratic questioning technique does not necessarily take more time than the use of closed questions; it is, perhaps, rather the opposite, because it may take many closed questions to get the same answer. Furthermore, you will often be more certain that the patient has said what he or she really wants thus avoid many of the so-called "doorknob questions" – "By the way …?" [147]. However, it may be appropriate sometimes to ask closed questions, e.g. if you have to be sure about the nature of a symptom.

Summaries
Summaries have proven to be a simple, but very effective method that may ensure that the patient feels understood. Summaries can be classified into three categories:

- **Repeating** the patient's own words, for example: "You say that you have periods of pain and that you felt depressed during those periods".
- **Rephrasing**, other words, but with the same meaning, e.g.: "It sounds like you are always depressed when you have pain".
- **Interpreting**, using different words, and giving the words a different meaning, e.g. "Can I understand you so that your symptoms make you depressed?"

While repeating the patient's experience and opinions, you may make sure that you have correctly understood the patient, and the patient will also feel heard and understood. This approach also serves to clarify (or reinforce) the patient's views and thus makes things more clear for the patient. It is something entirely different to hear it from someone else, even if it's your own words and opinion. Furthermore, many of the paradoxes or contradictions that may be in the patient's thinking will become apparent. When the patient becomes aware of such contradictions and the paradoxes, he or she will become curious paving the way for changes in thinking.

The summary may begin with phrases like: "Did I understand you correctly that you believe …?", "I want to be sure that I understood it correctly", "You are saying …", "If I have understood you correctly, then you are saying …", "I hear you say …", "On the one hand, … on the other hand, …". Finally, good summaries give an overview and give focus to the consultation process – both for the GP and the patient.

Express empathy (emotional feedback)
Showing empathy is a strong tool for making the patient feel heard and understood. This could be done by saying, "I can hear that it has been difficult for you (or caused you trouble)", "I can understand that it is uncomfortable for you", "I can see that you feel bad about… ". It is important to keep in mind that understanding and empathy are not tantamount to agreement with or acceptance of the patient's statements and actions. You may, for example, be critical of a patient's high consumption of pain medication from a medical perspective, while being empathetic to the patient's pain experience.

The techniques rope-a-dope and empowerment are discussed below, see the TERM Model step C.

Summary

Assessment techniques
1. Be conscious of your role and try to be proactive rather than reactive.
2. If possible, summarise previous illness episodes, reactions, patterns, psychiatric history and chronicity before the consultation (Table 11.1).
3. Throughout the assessment process, it is essential to use the Socratic questioning technique (neutral and genuine curiosity, open questions, encouragement) and to omit any explanations, corrections and lecturing (Table 11.2).
4. It is essential that the patient feels understood. Frequent summaries and empathy/emotional feedback should therefore be given.
5. Remember: The spirit is more important than the technique.

TERM model step A: Understanding

Table 11.3 features the various steps in the diagnostic assessment of patients who present functional symptoms. A systematic approach like this is also extremely useful for many other patients seen in the clinic. The model describes the consultation process, where step A is the patient's part, and where focus is on making the patient feel heard and understood.

Table 11.3 The TERM model

A. Understanding	
1.	Take a full symptom history (seek clarification, identify accompanying symptoms, describe a typical symptom day)
2.	Explore emotional cues.
3.	Inquire directly about symptoms of anxiety and depression.
4.	Explore stressors and external factors (social, work-related, and family).
5.	Explore functional level (physical, social, and family).
6.	Explore the patient's illness beliefs.
7.	Explore the patient's expectations to treatment and examination.
8.	Make a brief, focused physical examination and, if indicated, non-clinical examination.

B. The GP's expertise and acknowledgement	
1.	Provide feedback on the results of the physical examination.
2.	Acknowledge the reality of the symptoms.
3.	Make clear that there is no (or that there is indeed) indication for further examination or non-psychiatric treatment.

C. Negotiating a new or modified model of understanding	
1.	Clarify and modify the patient's illness understanding *The symptoms are put into alternative perspectives and the patient's illness understanding is nuanced.*
2.A.	Clarify possible and impossible causes – very important for the somatic specialist

2.B.	Mild cases
	a) Qualifying normalisation
	b) Reactions to strain, stress or nervousness
	  i) Palpitations when you get frightened
	  ii) More sensitive when depressed
	  iii) Muscular tension when frightened or nervous
	c) Demonstrate/present other possible associations
	  i) Practical (hyperventilation, muscular tension
	  ii) Link physical discomfort, emotional reactions and life events
	  iii) Here and now

2.C.   Severe cases
    a) Known phenomenon that has a name: *bodily distress syndrome* or functional disorder.
    b) Some people are more physically sensitive than others.
    c) Some people may produce more symptoms than others.
    d) How you react and respond to symptoms is important for how you will manage in the future (*coping*).

D. Summary and planning of follow-up

Summarise the contents of the day's consultation.
Negotiate objectives, contents and form of the further course with the patient:
1. Mild, transient cases → treatment is terminated.
2. Subacute cases → regular scheduled consultations.
3. Severe cases → consider status consultation with conversation therapy. Agree on regular scheduled consultations. See also management of chronic disorders.
4. Consider referral to psychiatrist, psychologist or specialist service.

E. Management of chronic disorders

A.1 Take a full symptom history

Even in cases where it is obvious that the patient does not have a well-defined physical disease that can explain the physical symptoms, it is important that the GP obtains a full symptom history and is insistent on getting the individual symptom clarified and specified as much as possible. The detailed knowledge of the patient's symptoms serves several purposes: 1) The patient feels heard concerning what matters most to him/her; 2) Both the GP and the patient get necessary insight into how the symptoms can vary; and 3) The GP's diagnosis rests on firmer ground, which allows the GP to speak with greater weight, even in the patient's eyes, about the lack of a basis for a possible physical ailment. Based on his expert knowledge, the GP will later be able to engage in an informed dialogue about the patient's concerns.

Patients with functional disorders may give so much focus to the suffering caused by their symptoms and to the negative consequences symptoms have for their lives and their quality of life that it may be difficult to obtain detailed insight into the nature of their symptoms. A thorough symptom review will therefore help the patients get an overview of their symptoms which may also seem confusing and frightening to the patients themselves. This alone can have a therapeutic effect.

It is also important to clarify whether the patient for some time has had several different symptoms and therefore maybe even meets the criteria for having a bodily distress syndrome. Questions could explore whether symptoms include cardio-pulmonary arousal, gastrointestinal arousal, musculoskeletal tension/pain and non-specific general symptoms, as shown in Table 4.2. The therapist may want to use a symptom checklist that the patient fills in or that informs the questions. As shown in the table, apart from a pattern of functional symptoms, a diagnosis is made on the basis of reduced functioning, i.e. the disease must be sufficiently debilitating to warrant a diagnosis by itself – otherwise the therapist may focus on the specific functional symptom for which the patient seeks help. A clinical picture dominated by excessive concern should invite questions about health anxiety (Table 4.4).

In order to obtain a concrete and detailed picture of the patient's symptoms, it may be very helpful to have the patient describe a "typical day with the symptom", for example yesterday. In more complicated cases, it may be useful to use a weekly symptom chart where the intensity and frequency, etc., of symptoms is recorded continuously at home by the patient (Appendix 1).

A.2 Explore emotional clues

The patients often narrate the difficulties they encounter because of their physical problems, e.g.: "I am so depressed about the fact that it does not go away", "if it doesn't soon becomes better, I'll take my own life". Without disputing or confirming causation, you may invite the patients to elaborate on how they feel and how they are: "Tell more about it", "You say that you feel the whole thing is confusing … (the patient's own words) – try to say something more about it (i.e. how you are)". Do not be hesitant to give emotional feedback, e.g.: "I understand that you are having a very difficult time". Or, ask openly: "What are your feelings about this?".

This approach allows you to talk about other things than physical symptoms, and it shifts the focus away and sends the signal that emotional factors may be relevant. Finally, patients will see this as an expression of a genuine interest in how they are. Attention should also be given to nonverbal signs of mental difficulty, and if this is the case, you may try to get it out into the open. You can, for example, say: "You appear to be tense, is this how you feel?".

A.3 Inquire directly about symptoms of anxiety and depression

Use general and open phrases and words such as, "How is your mood (by the way)", "How are your feelings about yourself?", "Are you able to relax?", "Are you feeling stressed?" Such phrases may be more acceptable than direct questions asking if the patient is depressed or anxious.

If the patient answers yes to these screening questions, he or she should be asked more direct questions about symptoms of depression and anxiety disorders, maybe using the psychometric screening forms, e.g. the Common Mental Disorder Questionnaire (CMDQ, Appendix 2).

A.4 Explore stressors and external factors (social, occupational and familial)

Functional symptoms may be a response to psychosocial stress. Similarly, the problems experienced by patients due to well-defined physical diseases may be exacerbated by stress or in stressful situations. Patients may be reluctant even to talk about such problems, because they believe that the GP only manages the physical problems. The patient will frequently have wondered whether there could be a connection, and the GP's unsolicited questions about such a connection will confirm to the patient that this may, indeed, be the case. If the patient suffers from a chronic condition, he may be particularly reluctant to mention thoughts about psychosocial factors to the GP because he will be afraid that the GP will then focus only on this dimension and not take seriously and thoroughly investigate his physical discomfort.

Examples of screening questions [181]:

+ Background: "What is (otherwise) happening in your life these days?"
+ Affect: "What are your feelings about this?"
+ Problems: "What is the biggest problem in this?"

- Handling: "How are you handling this?", "How have you coped with this?"
- Empathy: "It must be difficult for you".

Remember that it is important to enquire about the psychosocial situation at an early stage in the consultation process rather than to wait until all bio-medical aspects have been explored. Otherwise, the patient may interpret this as the GP's attempts to dismiss symptoms as something mental or social because he could find no biomedical cause.
[182]:

A.5 Explore functional level, handling of the illness (coping) and illness behaviour

The patients should be asked about the disruptions caused by their symptoms in terms of social functional capacity, including work and family relationship, for example: "How has this affected your ability to xx?", "How have you handled this?", "How have you previously handled this?". A systematic approach may take its starting point in the dimensions from the WHO Disability Assessment Schedule (WHO-DAS) [182]:

- Understanding and communication: "Are you able to concentrate on the things you do?"
- Mobility: "Are you able to move around – stand up – what is your maximal walking distance?"
- Personal hygiene: "What about getting dressed – are you able to wash yourself?", "How do you care for yourself during your everyday life?"
- Social competencies: "How is your contact with your friends and acquaintances?"
- Work: "How has this affected your work?"
- Household activities: "How are you managing your daily activities?"
- Outward activities: "To which extent do you participate in activities in the local community?"
- Incapacity: "How many days have you been reported absent from work over the past month? How many days have you been unable to make your usual chores?"

A.6 Explore the patient's illness beliefs
(and wait to tell your own)

In recent years, it has become clear that the patient's own illness perception and disease model are extremely important for morbidity and functional capacity, because they determine how the individual reacts to symptoms (see also Chapter 8 on disease understanding and symptom perception). It is therefore important to uncover the patient's illness perception.

- Identity: "What are your own thoughts about what is wrong with you?", "Have you thought about a particular disease?", "The symptoms you've described, do you think they are all caused by the same disease or are you thinking that you have multiple diseases?", "Are you not sure what is wrong with you, and what are your thoughts about this?".
- Cause: "What are your own thoughts about the cause of this?", "You must have thought something about what …", "Many people think about what is wrong and why they are feeling the way they are. What are your thoughts?", "Have you wondered why you got …?".
- Time horizon: "How long do you think it will last?", "Do you think it is a long-lasting or short-lived?".
- Consequences: "How do you think the symptoms will affect you?", "Which influence do you think it will have on your life, your daily life?", "Have you had thoughts that this could be something dangerous?".
- Control: "Have you thought about or do you have any experience of things that might improve or worsen your symptoms?".

If it is necessary, you may use one or few leading questions, as the patient may be reluctant to raise a subject in fear of the answer or in fear of appearing ignorant. It is essential to resist the temptation to correct the patient and interrupt to offer an explanation, even if it seems obvious to the GP. Instead, listen and ask out of interest, but do remember to maintain focus. REMEMBER that it is necessary to know the patient's mind in order to be able at a later stage to help the patient change this.

A.7 Explore the patient's expectations to the examination and treatment

Ask the patients about their expectations for their current visits. This helps uncover possible underlying reasons for the visit, including emotional elements, and it helps promote cooperation between the GP and the patient.

Knowledge of what the patient actually wants and expects will also make the GP better prepared to accommodate and respond to these expectations and more able to work towards a common consensus on treatment plan and goals.

Patients with functional disorders may have an unrealistic idea of the possibilities for (biomedical) treatment and the capability of science in terms of diagnosis, i.e. they do not have a realistic view of the limits of medical science (which also applies to some GPs). Patients may entertain the idea that there must be a demonstrable defect that could explain their symptoms and that "as long as the symptoms are investigated thoroughly enough, the GP will find out what is wrong and I'll be treated and get well". This may be one of the reasons that they frequently seek medical attention and maybe consult different GPs. Patients who have not accepted the limits of medicine may conclude that the GP will not examine or treat them properly. Ask the patient: "What are your thoughts about what should happen now?", "Have you thought about which investigations or treatments should be made?", "What are your expectations for coming here today?"

A.8 Make a focused clinical examination and any indicated paraclinical examinations

It has previously been a common misconception that you should avoid traditional objective investigation of patients with functional disorders in order not to give them a "secondary" benefit.

Patients with functional disorders are entitled to a proper investigation. But even in cases where the patient's symptom description does not raise suspicion of organ pathology, it might, for psychological reasons, be a good idea to perform a clinical examination of the relevant organ, e.g. auscultation of the heart if the patient complains of heart problems. This helps make the patient feel taken seriously and it shows that the GP cares. "According to what you tell me, it does not sound as if there is something seriously wrong with your heart, but if it is OK, I'd like to listen to it". If it is a repeated examination, then you might suggest that the indication is psychological: "I can see that you are worried, so I'd like to listen to your heart".

Particularly in patients with chronic disorders, the investigation should focus on clearly subjective complaints and objective findings (see Table 4.3); and in chronic functional disorders, investigations and tests should be avoided if they are not indicated by objective findings or a well-defined clinical disease picture.

TERM model step B: The GP's expertise and acknowledgement

B.1 Provide feedback on findings

Once the history has been taken and the patient has been clinically examined, the outcome should be summarised for the patient. It is important to mention both positive and negative findings. *You must not under any circumstances tell the patient that nothing is wrong.* However, you may say that the patient suffers neither from the disease that the patient thought about or feared, nor the disease that the GP investigated. You may, for example, say: "I have now examined your stomach (or any relevant body system), and I have found no signs of changes (that could explain your pain), or anything we may treat medically or surgically. You had a little soreness in your left side, which if often seen by muscle tension, and it is harmless".

It is important that you speak as a professional and demonstrate your expert knowledge based on observation, i.e. by "looking inside" the patient during the clinical examination, paraclinical test, etc. Feedback that uses this graphical metaphor may be communicated by phrases carrying the message that the GP has "seen into the patient", for example by spectroscopy or diagnostic imaging examinations. It is also important to give specific feedback. It carries more weight and is easier to understand for the patient if you say that you have "looked at the kidney and liver" using the blood samples, and that they are functioning as they should, than if you are simply saying "the blood tests are normal". Knowledge based on objective facts is a kind of knowledge the patient is neither able to possess nor to assess, and it thus cannot be challenged by the patient [142].

B.2 Acknowledge the reality of the symptoms

The GP may deliver the message that in his or her expert judgment, there are no signs of measurable organic or pathophysiological changes; yet, on the other hand, it is also important to recognise that the symptoms are genuine, because as a GP, you cannot dispute the fact that the patient <u>feels</u> ill and therefore is ill (i.e. the subjective experience of illness may prevail in the absence of any objective manifestation of medically verifiable disease or disorder). In this domain, the patient is the authority. Remarks inferring that the patient is not ill can be perceived as if the GP does not believe in the patient's symptoms, or suspects that the patient deliberately simulates.

The GP should therefore always acknowledge that the symptoms are real and you may, for example, say: "Fortunately, I can reassure you that there is no indication that this is a serious illness. But I can see you're very disturbed by your symptoms (e.g. pain)". It is important to realise that the patient's symptom experience is real, and that there may be neurobiological transformations even if they cannot be objectively measured in clinical routine investigations (see Chapter 6, "Biological mechanisms").

B.3 Explain that there is no indication for further tests or treatments

It should be made clear to the patient that based on the GP's expert knowledge and investigations (clinical, non-clinical, etc.), there is no basis for undertaking any further physical investigation or further diagnostic work-up, and that no resort can be made to any effective traditional medical or surgical treatments. This may discourage the patient from beginning to doubt whether a certain investigation was forgotten just after having left the clinic. The message also communicates to the patient that the decision to take no further action is rooted in the limits of medicine, not in the GP's unwillingness or lack of diligence: "I see no medical reason for any further investigations, and there is no surgical or medical treatment that will be able to help you". In your choice of words, it is important to take a starting point in the illness that the patient himself feared, or the treatment which he believed would help him.

TERM model step C

A common, basic assumption is that physical symptoms must be caused by a physical disease, i.e. organic changes or pathophysiological malfunctions – in spite of the fact that it has been demonstrated that it is more the exception than the rule that a physical symptom has a well-defined organic basis [32]. The either-or-idea is widespread: "If it is not something organic, it must be something mental". The latter is frequently equated with pure fantasy. This implies that the message communicated to the patient when the GP says that nothing organic is wrong is that the patient simply must "pull him- or herself together" or "stop right away". The implicit understanding is that the situation is created by the patient and it is therefore the patient's own fault.

If the patient feels that others, especially the GP, believe that it is his/her own fault, any treatment is virtually impossible. The patient will feel rejected and powerless and will not know what to do [183]. The patient, rightly, cannot understand this. It is therefore essential that the patient be helped to see the illness in a more nuanced and realistic perspective. The goal is to help the patient understand the illness, to convey that the patient is not to blame, and that one can do something oneself and can obtain some control over the symptoms/illness (empowerment). The aim is thus to reframe the complaints, i.e. place them in new contexts, and to give the patient an expanded understanding and an alternative model of understanding. As previously mentioned, it is very important that the patient does not feel that he/she is being corrected, and it is exceedingly effective if the patient can reach some of the conclusions him- or herself.

It is essential that an explanation suggested by the GP does not collide with the patient's own understanding; if this appears to be the case, a slower-paced process should be used. Try to get several possible explanations on the table, even if the patient is dismissive. If this appears to be the case, it is crucial to uncover the patient's own understanding and perceptions.

Before explaining step C of the model (C in Table 11.3), some more essential conversation techniques will be presented.

General conversation techniques

Avoid conflict

In some cases, it is not possible to alter the patient's belief in a specific organic basis for the complaints, and it is important not to get into a locked and confrontational discussion. Conflicts are often caused by misapprehensions. Bend to the argument or go with the patient's resistance; (with a professional boxing expression called *rope-a-dope*). The patient may, for example, suspect that he has heart disease in which case the GP may say, "I can hear (or see) that you are convinced that there must be something wrong with your heart (or another organ)", "I cannot find any sign of change in your heart, and therefore there is nothing we can treat surgically or medically to make the symptoms disappear. On the other hand, there are several things you can do to get better, which had also been the case if we had found an actual heart disease. What do you think; should we talk about this?" Depending on the nature of the problem, you should then become very concrete, for instance: "You know that exercise is important to avoid getting worse. This also applies to people with heart disease. How does this sound to you?", "Many people are afraid that the heart would be damaged if they exercised, or that it might even kill you. Is this something you've thought about?", "What do you think will happen if you start to exercise?", "I can reassure you that it will not happen. However, I can say with certainty that you will get worse if you do not exercise – it is important that you keep yourself going, although I understand that it may be difficult for you". It is important that this process takes the form of a negotiation with the patient.

Support self-help and own control (empowerment)

It is very important to support the patient's feeling of being able to do something and to have control over his illness and symptoms. This can be achieved by practical demonstrations and by helping the patient get a new understanding of his disease and what is going on in general. This approach is also called *empowerment* or *self-efficacy*. *Empowerment* means power, force and strength, where growth in knowledge, insight and self-awareness goes hand in hand with drive. *Empowerment* is also closely associated with patient satisfaction [183].

Contrary to what we as GPs are often tempted to believe, the patient sees himself, and not the GP, as the highest authority. The GP is perceived more as a consultant, who is often in competition with alternative therapists, the internet, magazines, friends, family, etc. [184]. The patient can use the GP to test his hypotheses and thoughts about a relation or to get confirmation of the correctness of his ideas. If you want to effect changes in the patient, the new ideas must therefore fit into the patient's mind and be tested and accepted by the patient, i.e. by the final authority. Using the summation technique, this may be achieved by letting the patient voice his own solutions and by gently guiding the patient by emphasising, underscoring and focusing select elements of the summary. It is important that the patient does not feel that you reject his interpretations, but that he is taken seriously. Ideally, the conversation should take the form of a dialogue between the GP and the patient. ….". You may communicate recognition of the patient's thoughts with utterances like: "I do understand your thinking".

TERM model step C: Negotiation of a new or modified model of understanding

C.1 Clarify the patient's illness beliefs

The patient told about his illness and illness behaviour when the diagnostic assessment took place. The patient's illness perceptions are now further clarified (see also Table 8.1), and the GP makes sure that all possible (and impossible) causal explanations have been raised. Any causal explanations that the GP believes the patient may not have given or that the GP thinks may be relevant (e.g. mental or social stressors) are suggested to the patient and may be included in the negotiation. Possible explanatory models to which the GP may resort are explained below. The goal is to help the patient see the symptoms in alternative contexts and to give him a more nuanced understanding of his illness.

C.2.A Clarify possible and impossible causal explanations

The somatic specialist is in a unique position within his area of specialisation to respond to the patient's ideas about what can be wrong, and clarifying which causal explanations are possible and which are not will be of much help in the later course. This should be a natural part of any diagnostic process.

The evidence and professional knowledge available within the specialty should be communicated to the patient in a manner that can be duly incorporated into the examination of possible causal explanations and behaviour. Working with the patient's understanding of his disease can sometimes be a lengthy process that requires more follow-up conversations (see pp. 124-6 "Follow-up conversations").

C.2.B Treatment of mild cases

C. 2.B. a Qualifying normalisation and reassurance

All people have daily physical sensations. Physical sensations are thus entirely normal – and a way in which the body sends a signal about its current state. We may thus see this as a sense that helps protect the body against injury and stress. We do not know precisely why some are more burdened by physical sensations/symptoms than others. When the GP uses normalisation and reassurance, it is important that he takes as his point of departure the patient's expressed concerns and illness understanding. Failing to do so, the GP will not reach the patient and the treatment will not have the intended effect [185]. "I can hear that you are afraid that the rumbling and 'uneasiness' in your stomach could be due to a gastric ulcer. However, I can reassure you that it is something quite normal, and most people sometimes have it; it is not a sign of a gastric ulcer".

C. 2.B.b Reaction to strains, stress or nervousness

It should be mentioned that it is entirely normal sometimes to have physical symptoms in response to stress and strain, and/or that existing physical symptoms may get worse. Physical symptoms are only rarely caused by organic or pathophysiological dysfunction, e.g.: "All people may react with physical symptoms and discomfort when having problems or feeling pressured or stressed", "It is not dangerous, but I can understand it worries you and is uncomfortable", "I often see these symptoms in people who are stressed or tense. Could this also be true of you?". In some cases, the patient may have a hard time believing it.

In the patient's mind, this change of perspective on the cause of the symptoms may be very radical, and you must therefore give the patient time to process this information. This is done best by letting the patient make suggestions and voice his thoughts and by helping the patient to weigh the pros against the cons.

Examples of simple explanations could be:

- You may experience palpitations, shortness of breath and other physical symptoms when frightened or nervous about something. Most patients have experienced this and may give their own examples.
- You are more sensitive to physical symptoms when you are depressed.
- You tighten your muscles when you become anxious or stressed. This may cause pain, which, in turn, may increase the tension and cause more pain, so you are trapped in a vicious circle.

C. 2. B.c Demonstration/presentation of possible associations

Muscle ache can be demonstrated, for example, by asking the patient to hold a book with his arm stretched out, which almost always leads to pain after some time: Even a slight muscle tone will cause the muscle to ache in a short time. Logically, an even poorer muscle tonus should therefore give rise to muscle ache when the tonus persists almost around the clock. In some cases, tension headache may be demonstrated by pressing the patient's tense neck muscles.

Examples from everyday life and practical exercises can be powerful tools for demonstrating the connection between physical symptoms, feelings and behaviour. Furthermore, it is very important that the demonstrations give the patient the experience that he may influence the symptoms and that they are not entirely beyond his control. It is often possible to establish a connection between emotional reactions and life events that involve physical reactions. The patient is gradually guided into talking about problems related to straining and stressful events. It is most effective to use the patient's own examples: "You told me before that you were particularly ill last Monday. It was also the day you told me that your husband had come home very late. I was wondering if there might be a connection? What do you think?" Finally, here-and-now situations may arise spontaneously. "I can see it makes you feel bad when we talk about this. How is your stomach right now?" The patient has often been nervous about the visit to the GP, and you may check whether this has caused the physical symptoms to become worse.

C.2.C Treatment of severe cases

In more severe cases of functional disorders where a pathological disorder may be present, the simple techniques will not be sufficient. The use of normalisation, in particular, will fail in these cases. However, it is still necessary to give the patient a meaningful understanding of his illness.

C. 2.C.a The disorder is known and has a name
The patients often think that they are the only ones in the world who have this disease and are therefore afraid that they are the only ones in whom something has been missed. They must therefore be informed that their illness is a known phenomenon that has a name: functional disorder or *bodily distress syndrome* (or another relevant name). An example of a phrasing might be: "There are many who suffer from the same illness as you, so it's definitely not uncommon", "We also have a name for it; we call it a functional disorder or bodily distress syndrome (or another name, such as bodily state of stress or chronic pain disorder)". The patient will then typically ask what it is.

C.2.C.b-c Cause unknown but possible biological basis
You may then continue by explaining that the fundamental cause is unknown, like in many other diseases (e.g. essential hypertension). For example, you may say that: "Actually, we do not know the cause or mechanism behind this, but a lot of research is going on", "We know with great certainty that it is not due to some hidden physical disease, and we know that neither traditional medical nor surgical treatment helps, but may, instead, exacerbate the illness".

There is growing evidence that biological factors play a role in the disease process, and to free the patient from feeling guilt, the possibility of biological reasons should be mentioned (similarly, we are now quite sure that there is a biological substrate in depression). You may, for example, say: "Several studies suggest that the cause may be some changes in the brain, and some people are more physically sensitive than others and they are, so to say, not so good at filtering out physical sensations and symptoms and are therefore more troubled by symptoms. In some people, the body also produces more symptoms, just as if you e.g. become frightened and your heart begins to beat faster (see also Chapter 5, "Aetiology"). In other cases, other examples may be used. We all know the phenomenon that when we hear about or come to think of fleas and lice, we begin to scratch our hair because it itches: Senses and awareness are heightened. In functional disorders, sensitivity is just much higher. In addition, you may mention that "we know that in some people, heredity also plays a role".

C. 2.C.d Coping – the importance of behaviour regardless of cause
Coping plays an important role in many kinds of illnesses because it influences the extent to which a disease affects the individual's ability to function and his quality of life and thus the prognosis of the disease. Our illness behaviour and social illness behaviour are determined by the thoughts and ideas we have about our illness. A certain behaviour may seem incomprehensible to the GP, but it may be a perfectly logical and rational behaviour in light of the patient's perception of the problem. It may be difficult for the patient to understand why his behaviour is an issue because he thinks that it is due to his illness, and he sees no other options. You may use phrases such as: "How you act upon and react to your symptoms is important for how you will be in the future – this is true for all diseases", "Two pairs of eyes see more than one pair, and together we may come up with some suggestions you never thought could be an option". "It is important that you do what you can to function as well as possible despite the difficulties you are experiencing". "It is all about developing new coping strategies and stopping strategies that do no good or are harmful". "You've seen many GPs and tried several treatments and investigations that did not work". "One thing is certain – it will not help you if you expose yourself to unnecessary investigations or treatments (acceptance of the limits of medicine)".

TERM model step D: Summary and planning of further treatment course

The result of the consultation should be summarised at the end, e.g. you may ask the patient: "How have you benefited from our conversation?", "Is there anything you can use?", "Would it be reasonable to do (so and so)?", "Can we agree on ...?". In some cases – especially in chronic cases – is not it possible to change the patient's perception of the cause of the complaints, and it is important that you do not engage in a locked and confrontational discussion. Instead of sticking to a discussion of causality, you may suggest to the patient that you try to find out whether the way he/she manages her everyday life and some of the things he/she is doing are aggravating or improving his/her condition – i.e. shift the focus from illness perception to behaviour and coping.

The further treatment course must thus be **negotiated** with the patient. You may argue that there are other options for treatment than those that are purely medical or surgical. You may suggest that you jointly find out if this appeals to the patient. Suggest that you and the patient together explore what he/she can do to get better, no matter what the cause of the problem is.

The following four courses should be considered (see also Chapter 9 and Figure 9.1 *Stepped care* and Chapter 12):

1. Mild cases: Qualifying normalisation and termination of treatment.
2. Moderate cases: Agree on follow-up treatment in the form of a series of conversations with fixed times and intervals.
3. Severe/chronic cases: A status consultation. Agree on consultations at fixed times and intervals.
4. Possibly referral to a psychiatrist, psychologist with special expertise in this area or specialist centre.

TERM model step E: Management of chronic disorders

In the most severe cases, the chronic functional disorder is a lifelong condition where the patient can be severely impaired. In many of these cases, it is therefore more realistic to talk about coping or management than about cure. This means that the therapeutic strategy should not aim to cure the patient; rather, it should aim at giving the patient the best possible life with his/her illness, just as in any other chronic physical diseases and mental disorders.

You may often feel insecure about the patient with a chronic illness since you have no overview of all the examinations and treatments the patient has gone through and the various syndromes the patient has presented. The typical picture will be one of a mixture of possible positive findings and obvious functional somatic symptoms. The patient will be no less confused. The practitioner may think: "Is it her again, what should I do? Could I have overlooked something in her extensive medical history?". You feel insecure about seeing the patient and must pull yourself together when seeing the patient in the waiting room. A good way of obtaining an overview of and get to grips with the management of a chronic functional disorder is to agree on a status consultation.

It is important in complex cases or in patients with chronic functional disorders to be conscious of your own role in the treatment, i.e. where is the most appropriate place to treat the patient, and is this possible (see Figure 9.1). It is rarely a good idea to treat patients with functional disorders in the secondary health care system – except in the case of certain multidisciplinary care facilities like back care centres.

The task of the specialist unit is thus to terminate its own treatment of the patient in a manner that allows others to continue the treatment course. Even in specialised units, it may be necessary to familiarise oneself with complex cases, which requires knowledge of the treatment of chronic cases.

Status consultation

Before the consultation
Allocate the necessary time to review the patient's case. In certain cases, it may seem overwhelming and require time and effort, but the effort pays off later, both in terms of saved time and in the relationship with the patient.

Summary

Before the status consultation

- Allocate the necessary time to review the patient's case.
- Review the patient's medical history based on medical records, discharge summaries, etc.
- Summarise the symptom pictures the patient has presented and for which examinations have been performed into a few main categories or themes.
- Summarise the examinations and treatments the patient has been through – possibly for each cluster of symptoms, including positive and negative findings.
- Look for any patterns in illness severity over time and complaints in relation to external stress and events in the patient's life.
- Look for signs of mental disorders.

Review the patient's medical history based on patient records, discharge summaries, etc. *Summarise the symptom pictures* the patient has presented and for which examinations have been performed into (few) major groups. *Summarise the evaluation and treatment* the patient has been through, including positive and negative findings. Making such a statement of no more than 1-2 pages with a few major points will give a clearer picture and you may feel on safer ground. It is important that both negative and positive findings are included so that the patient does not feel that one half of the picture has been left out. Please also *note any possible patterns* in degrees of illness over time and complaints in relation to external pressures and events that the patient has experienced.

Look for psychiatric disorders. Physical and emotional symptoms often occur simultaneously and worsen simultaneously. In a depression, the patient can focus solely on the physical symptoms which may previously have disappeared with the treatment of depression. This correlation can be made clear to the patient and instigate a conversation on the subject.

Summary

During the status consultation

+ Tell the patient about the background of the status consultation.
+ Provide the summary of the medical history as neutral facts. For example, "read" the record together with the patient.
+ Explore the patient's expectation to the healthcare system. On this basis, conclude that traditional medical treatment (alone) will fall short.
+ Offer the patient that you together try to find out how the patient can get better.
+ Apply general conversation techniques and offer general counsel for chronic functional disorders.

During the consultation

Explain the background for the status consultation to the patient. You may explain to the patient that he/she has gone through many examinations and treatments that have not really helped, that he/she has often been to the clinic, that he/she is very troubled, and that you can see that he/she is having a difficult time. You do not feel that you are getting anywhere with the traditional medical treatment. You will now try to look at it with new eyes, because it is hardly satisfactory with all the examinations and examinations that do not help. You may for example say to the patient: "Shouldn't we see if we could help each other find a new way, so that you can get better?", "Sadly, there are many diseases we cannot treat so that they go away completely, but we can do something to make you feel better", "There is no miracle cure", "One goal could be to stop unnecessary examinations that do not help anyway", "I will, of course, look out for any signs of physical disease you may get".

Present the summary of the *disease history as neutral facts.* It is important that both positive and negative findings are highlighted and discussed with the patient. It is also important that the GP is meticulous when providing the somatic review and that it is made absolutely clear to the patient that he/she can be sure that the GP will look out for new physical disease if new symptoms occur. The summing up and the resulting overview helps not only the GP get an overview, but will also be for the benefit of the patients and, if desired, their families, which have often been through a long and chaotic trajectory.

The limits of medicine (medical science)

GPs must acknowledge that only a small part of physical symptoms are rooted in morbidity and disability that may be explained on the basis of the biomedical model, and we are able to treat an even smaller part of these symptoms. Many GPs and patients have not realised this, and it may be one reason why patients with functional disorders continue to seek treatment. It should be noted that this applies not only to functional disorders, but also to many physical diseases. Essential hypertension may be seen as an analogous example – the treatment goals in this disorder are also to avoid secondary damage.

Besides the GP being conscious of the limits of medical science, it is important that the GP actively inquires about the patient's expectations to treatment (see Section A.7, TERM Model).

General advice on management of chronic functional disorders

The following general advice applies in the management of chronic functional disorders (see also Table 11.4):

1-3: Perform a *physical examination* that focuses on the organ system the patient complains about. This helps the patient feel taken seriously and not superficially treated. Throughout the examination and in the entire assessment of the patient, it is important to *emphasise objective findings* instead of subjective complaints. *Avoid diagnostic assessment and assessments* that are not indicated by objective findings or a well-defined (new) clinical pathology. In chronic functional disorders, the probability is a very small (<1-2%) that you will eventually find a disease that may explain the disease [17,132,134]. On the other hand, patients with functional disorders are just as likely as other people to get an (independent) genuine physical disease.

4: *Rationalise medication. Avoid addictive medication.* The typical patient with a functional disorder takes several different kinds of medication. Consider whether the medication, both psychoactive and other types, are doing more harm than good. Some patients with functional disorders have a significant potential for misuse. The drug may cause physical damage and it is expensive for the patient who often becomes psychologically dependent and may use it as evidence of his illness to his surroundings and himself. The patient will often resist any rationalisation of their medication. It is important to explain the cause of the changes. "You've been taking this medication for a while now and I can see that it has not really helped you because you continue to have symptoms. I therefore think we should try to gradually phase out this medication". Warn the patient that this may involve discomfort during a transitional period. It may be more difficult to phase out psychoactive and analgesic medication. You may try to explain: "I can hear that you are afraid to give up the medication and that you feel that it helps you somewhat. I'm sure that once you get used to not taking the medicine, you will get better as it also dulls you and you can get addicted to it so that you get more problems than you already have. This medicine helps only in the short term". Be firm, but not tough or punitive when phasing out the medication. Prevention is better than cure, so it is better to avoid potentially addictive medicines.

5: Make the diagnosis and tell the patient that the disorder is known and has a name. The diagnosis is also important because keeping this in mind makes you think very carefully before ordering new tests or treatments (see sections 1-3). Furthermore, something unknown is often associated with anxiety and uncertainty both for doctors and patients. When "the enemy gets a face" and a name, it becomes easier for the patient (and the doctor) to handle it and to deal with it. This reduces anxiety [158].

6: Acknowledge the reality of the patient's symptoms. The importance of this cannot be overemphasised since it will be a prerequisite for gaining the patient's acceptance and cooperation.

7: Be direct and honest with the patient about what you agree with and what you disagree with, but avoid that the patient feels stupid, put down or not respected. Please show respect. "I can hear that you are finding it difficult to believe what I am saying".

8: Be stoic, expect no quick changes or cure. Hold back for some time before you judge whether a treatment has helped or not.

9: Reduce the expectations to healing and accept the patient as chronically ill, but also support the belief that the patient can get better. The goal is to be able to contain the patient and his/her problems (*containment*) and to limit (iatrogenic) harm. It is thus a question more of management than of treatment in the same way as with other chronic physical and mental disorders.

10: Consider whether new symptoms or an exacerbation of already known symptoms reflect a worsening of the functional state and possibly a current stress situation rather than signs of a new physical disease. Knowing the patient, you could, for instance, say: "Nothing you said makes me think that you have contracted a new disease", "We've previously discussed that you have a strong bodily response to events, and I was wondering if something has happened recently or if there is something special that concern you now?"

11-12: Try, for example, a specific therapy (see TERM Model steps A-C and Part III on follow-up conversations) and consider referral to specialised treatment if any such is available.

13-15: Psychopharmacological treatment. Controlled trials of the effects of various psychoactive substances in functional disorders are few, but some evidence does exist that antidepressants, especially broad-spectrum ones, have some effect [23, 24, 26, 161,177,178]. However, it is important to switch medicines or taper any medicine that has no effect when a drug has been used in sufficient dosage and for a sufficient time (see also 'Pharmacological treatment', p. 78 and Table 9.1 p. 72).

16: Treat any other mental disorder according to the usual guidelines. In the chronic cases, more than 50% of the patients with functional disorders also have a mental disorder. Start at smaller doses than usual, and increase the dose more slowly because patients with functional disorders often have both a low threshold and a low tolerance for side effects. Be stoic and try to stick to any treatment that has been initiated until the patient has completed a sufficient treatment course. Preferably choose medication that can be monitored by serum analysis to take account of the fact that these patients can be very unstable in their drug habits and in their compliance, and because you avoid being dependent on the patient's subjective information about side effects.

17: Be conscious of your role in the treatment. If you see the patient in your capacity as a specialist, you should evaluate your role in the treatment. The patient may have a somewhat different view of the problem and the former treatment than the medical professional(s) who undertook such treatments), so you should always speak with the primary doctor(s) before doing anything that could intervene in existing treatment plans. Try to find out how you may best support the primary therapist in your capacity as a specialist and make sure always to coordinate treatments. It is a great advantage to think in a *stepped care* model, both to clarify your own role and to ensure a coherent treatment course.

18-19: Be proactive instead of reactive. Negotiate a series of consultations with fixed appointments at 2-6-week intervals (which may be supplemented with one phone consultation per week) and avoid consultations at the patient's request. This is an absolute prerequisite for any treatment or management of patients with functional symptoms of a certain duration and severity level.

20: If the patient has a job, any sick-listing should be avoided if at all possible. Patients with functional disorders can be inclined to be engulfed in their sick role and to enter into self-perpetuating vicious circles where they feel confirmed in how bad they are and how little they can manage. It is important to articulate the reason for not sick-listing the patient in a way that does not make the patient feel rejected or not understood. The risk associated with a short-term sick leave is probably negligent if a patient with a functional disorder suffers physical trauma, like a bone fracture. This can be explained by the clinical observation that patients can distinguish between genuine disease and functional symptoms, although they are not conscious of this distinction [17].

21: If you have primary responsibility for the patient's treatment, you should try to become the patient's only doctor and limit the patient's contact with other therapists, doctors and alternative therapists as much as possible. The healthcare system (and the grey market, etc.) has a significant share of the responsibility for chronification and iatrogenic harm in patients with functional disorders who are often treated and diagnosed in the same way as patients with genuine physical disease. Many investigations and treatments may be associated with a significant risk of physical damage and involve both human and economic costs for the patient. Talk with the patient about it and create an alliance.

22: Tell your colleagues about your treatment plan and make arrangements with your colleagues if you take time off. Doctors who do not know the patient may often fall short when encountering patients with severe functional disorders because their history is often confusing and the patient presents his own understanding. It is therefore important that colleagues have the necessary information and any instructions to treat the patient properly and to withstand the patient's pressure that something ought to be done here and now.

23: Attempt to build a therapeutic alliance with the patient's relatives by informing them about the treatment plan. In patients with chronic functional disorders in particular, there is often a very close symbiotic interaction within the family. In many cases, the whole family's life centres around the patient and his or her disease, and changes can be directly counteracted by family due to misunderstandings or because they may upset a fragile balance of power in the family. Changes will therefore interfere deeply in the whole family's life, and it can be a very complex matter to change such patterns. It is mandatory that the family is in agreement with or – even better – will support the patient in undergoing treatment and the necessary behavioural changes. Family therapy per se requires specialised knowledge, but it is always possible to arrange a consultation with the patient and his family. You may wish to consider soliciting domestic support or any similar help, including help from the local psychiatric team, if possible.

24: Arrange any necessary support/supervision for yourself if you are the primary care provider. Patients with chronic functional disorders may be some of the most difficult patients to treat and manage. In some cases, the doctor is exposed to almost constant pressure to undertake examinations and initiate physical treatment. Because patients can be very active in their search for treatment, many other therapists may try to interfere in the treatment and suggest inappropriate treatments or offer unnecessary explanations because of their lack of knowledge of the patient. Therefore, it is a good idea to have a colleague with whom you may discuss the problems.

Table 11.4 General advice on management of patient with chronic functional disorders

Physical
1. Make a physical examination focusing on the organ system from which the patient has (new) complaints.
2. Avoid assessment and treatment, unless indicated by objective signs or a well-defined (new) clinical illness picture
3. Never treat a patient for an illness he or she does not have.
4. Reduce unnecessary drugs, do not use on-demand prescriptions, and avoid habit-forming medication.

Psychological
5. Make the diagnosis and tell the patient that the disorder is known and has a name.
6. Acknowledge the reality of the patient's symptoms.
7. Be direct and honest with the patient about the areas you agree on and those you do not agree on, but be careful as not to make the patient feel ignorant, humiliated or not respected.
8. Be stoic; do not expect rapid changes or cures.
9. Reduce expectations to cure and accept that the patient suffers from a chronic disorder, but make sure to support the patient in believing that he will get better. The objective is to accept the patient and limit (iatrogenic) harm.
10. Consider if worsening of symptoms or appearance of new ones is a possible worsening of the functional disorder rather than a sign of new disease.
11. Consider trying a specific therapy and consider referral to specialist treatment.
12. Motivate the patient to accept specialized psychiatric treatment if relevant and available.

Psychopharmacological treatment
13. Consider treatment with psychoactive drugs (primarily antidepressants and, secondly, antiepileptics).
14. Avoid habit-forming mediation and, if possible, choose medication that can be serum monitored.
15 Start with a smaller dosage than usual and increase slowly. Be stoic about side effects.
16. Treat any coexisting psychiatric disorder according to usual guidelines.

Administrative

17. Be conscious of your role in the treatment
18. Be proactive rather than reactive if you are the patient's primary health care provider. Schedule a series of appointments of a fixed duration and with fixed intervals instead of leaving the scheduling to the patient's discretion.
19. Contact the patient's primary health care provider, often a general practitioner, and arrange treatment/diagnostic assessment if you are not his primary health care provider yourself.
20. If the patient has a job, sick leave should be avoided if at all possible.
21. Try to make an alliance with the patient so that you become the patient's only doctor, and minimize the patient's contact to other health care professionals, out-of-hours services and alternative therapists.
22. Inform your colleagues about your treatment plan and make arrangements with your colleagues if you take a day off.
23. Try to build an alliance with the patient's relatives by informing them about the treatment plan.
24. Arrange any necessary support/follow-up for yourself.

PART III

FOLLOW-UP TREATMENT

CHAPTER 12

Follow-up treatment

PER FINK, MARIANNE ROSENDAL, TOMAS TOFT AND ANDREAS SCHRÖDER

As stated in Chapter 9 (see Figure 9.1) and the TERM Model step E (Table 11.3), the treatment follows a stepped care principle where treatment is tailored to the severity of the illness. This section offers a brief overview of the follow-up treatment that can be arranged for mild, moderate and severe cases.

Mild cases with functional somatic symptoms

Any discomfort will probably lie within the normal range if the patient suffers from a mild disorder and if the patient's history contains no information about moderate to severe functional disorders. After having used the general model during the consultation and the symptoms have been "normalised", as stated in the TERM Model Step C. 2. B (Table 11.3), the treatment should be terminated. In individual cases, it may be appropriate to agree that the patient can return if needed.

Moderate functional disorders

Patients with acute functional symptoms are those who come back or have previously contacted the clinic because of functional symptoms, but if the problem has been present for less than 6 months, it may prove expedient to suggest follow-up treatment. Agree on a short series of regularly scheduled appointments. If the GP already masters a particular method or technique, this may be used in combination with elements from the TERM

Model. The next chapter will describe other options. Furthermore, the advice offered in the chapter on chronic functional disorders (see Chapter 11, Table 11.6) may also be applied in the treatment of patients with a shorter illness duration.

Severe functional disorders

Like in other chronic disorders, these patients need care tailored to their chronic condition. It is important that both the patient and the GP perceive the practitioner as a stable and lifelong coordinator and partner. The importance of consultations at fixed intervals cannot be emphasised strongly enough. Please see Chapter 11 step E for the treatment and management of chronic functional disorders and Chapter 13.

Referral to a specialist

The possibilities for referral vary according to local circumstances. The best is, of course, if the GP has a competent colleague who is a psychiatrist with whom to discuss the patient (*shared care*), but referral may be necessary in some cases. Unfortunately, general psychiatry rarely undertakes the diagnostic assessment or treatment of this group, and there are only few specialised units, if any, in most countries around the world.

Some patients may have difficulty understanding why they should be referred to a psychiatrist – because they believe that they are struggling with a physical problem. It is therefore necessary to explain the rationale to the patient in an empathetic way. An example of how to articulate a reason for a referral may be: *"I am glad to say that we have ruled out the possibility that your symptoms are caused by a serious bodily disorder. However, I understand that your pain (or other symptom) is still a big problem. The problems you have at home and how tense they make you worries me, and this definitely not contributing toward making you feel better. I have a colleague, who is a psychiatrist, who is interested in chronic pain (or another symptom) and who often gives me advice about patients with this kind of problem. I would therefore appreciate hearing his opinion about the best way to proceed"* [135].

CHAPTER 13

Contents of the follow-up treatment

PER FINK, ANDREAS SCHRÖDER AND MARIANNE ROSENDAL

The following is not intended as a treatment model, but rather as a tool box where you may pick your own favourites or whatever best fits a given problem. The treatments and interviewing techniques, as described in the TERM Model in Chapter 11, may also be used during the follow-up treatment, but this Chapter describes some additional methods and tools for further treatment.

Like in all other therapies, this therapy is taught through practical exercises and training. We therefore recommend that you attend courses or training rather than train and learn through self-study. Chapter 14 will also provide a proposal on how a brief psychological treatment in primary care may be planned and conducted.

Cognitive behavioural therapy has provided the best evidence in terms of improved patient function, reduced consumption of health services and increased quality of life in patients with chronic functional disorders [25;58;161;175]. The TERM Model is largely based on cognitive therapy. It should be mentioned, however, that cognitive therapy is not a unique therapy, but rather one that consists of a range of basic principles. Cognitive therapy for functional disorders is closely tailored to this patient group. A large number of therapists today offer cognitive behavioural therapy, but few therapists master the specific techniques that are necessary in functional disorders.

It can be useful to integrate into primary care both elements from the general principles of cognitive behavioural therapy as well as the more specialised techniques applied in functional disorders [160]. In addition to cognitive behavioural therapy (CBT), substantial evidence supports the use of graded exercise. In addition, techniques such as problem-solving and coping strategies designed for use in primary care may be deployed.

Follow-up consultations

If and to which extent the GP should schedule follow-up consultations with the patient depends on the GP's role in the treatment. The non-psychiatric medical specialist will usually not be involved in the subsequent treatment, but in rare cases it may be appropriate to schedule follow-up consultations. The medical or surgical specialist has a special position in terms of modifying the patient's own perception of the problem. Any dysfunctional beliefs about his illness (cause, nature, treatment, etc.) may hinder appropriate patient treatment, and with his professional authority, the specialist doctor is well placed to modify or alter such patient beliefs. Moreover, the patient may simultaneously have both a physical disease that demands treatment and functional symptoms, so it may be expedient that the specialist follows the patient. The general practitioner is often the patient's primary doctor and is therefore in a natural position, if he/she has the requisite qualifications, to assume responsibility for any follow-up consultations with the patient.

Table 13.1 Follow-up consultations

In general
• Current, specific and concrete problems. Not childhood or past.
• Conversation is dialogue.
• Set a fixed duration (e.g. 10, 20 el. 30 min.), and keep to schedule.
• Help the patient solve the problem, i.e. negotiate.
• The patient himself makes the choice.
• Discuss and schedule an appointment for termination of the treatment well ahead of termination, preferably with two or three consultations to go.

Follow-up consultations – general aspects

You should not neglect hearing about the patient's physical symptoms, but, on the other hand, be careful that this does not take up too much time during your encounter. The patient's need to talk about his/her symptoms will often subside as the treatment progresses. Instead, you should focus on the factors that cause the problems and help maintain the patient's symptoms and behaviours. GPs should also be wary of their own tendency to talk about or raise the issue of physical symptoms. The conversation should normally address current, specific and concrete issues, not the childhood or the past which may be better dealt with through regular psychotherapy (Table 13.1). Dealing with childhood can be relevant in long-term psychotherapy, but it is rarely a good idea in other situations, rather the contrary. The patient who has many "skeletons in his cupboard" can become completely absorbed and paralysed. Such a patient will find it very helpful to be held firmly in the present and in practical, concrete issues. For other patients, talking about their childhood can be an escape from dealing with their current problems.

Conversation as therapy follows a defined structure, as listed in Table 13.2. The structure maintains focus and ensures progress in therapy.

Conversation is a dialogue. As previously emphasised, it is important to always ensure that you have a common understanding with the patient and that you use the Socratic interviewing technique. The goal is through negotiation to help the patient solve the problems him/herself. It is the patient him/herself who ultimately chooses which problem areas should be confronted.

Arrange a **termination date** well in advance, preferably 2-3 conversations before termination. Once an end date has been agreed upon, the dialogues will automatically change character and become more far-sighted ("How do I cope with new problems in the future – from whom can I expect help?" etc.).

Table 13.2 The structure of a therapy session

Every session should have a fixed schedule

1. Make an agenda and choose which topics should be raised.
2. Schedule an appointment for the next session (may be omitted if appointments have already been made for several sessions).
3. What happened since you last met?
4. Go through any home assignments.
5. Work with specific techniques (problem, thought, behaviour, task, etc.).
6. Agree on home assignments.
7. Talk about things that may prevent the patient from doing home assignments and what may help the patient do the assignment.
8. Summarise the therapy session and the agreements you have made.

Problem-solving model

Problem-solving is a simple technique developed for use in primary care (Table 13.3). It is useful in many contexts and for different kinds of problems, and you may say that it is the backbone of almost all forms of therapy. Problem-solving therapy has proven effective and is easily applicable for the treatment of functional disorders in primary care [188;189]. The method is suitable for helping the patient in a structured way and in a few sessions to explore and solve problems that have proven difficult for the patient to handle. The patient learns to use his/her own skills and experience to handle both present and future problems.

The GP acts more as a consultant and trainer than as an expert. A problem-solving session generally lasts more than the 10-12 minutes usually allocated for a consultation in primary care [9], so it is recommended to use a regular therapy session. Since it is impossible for the patient (and the therapist) to address the entire complex of problems in one session, you may treat only one problem at a time. Always start by setting an agenda and review the outcome of any tasks solved since the last session. Appendix 3 offers a problem-solving table that can be used with the patient.

Table 13.3 Problem-solving technique

The eight steps in the problem-solving model are followed step by step:

1. Identify and narrow down a current problem, e.g. that the patient keeps to him/herself and does not go out.
2. Clarify any alternative objectives and define one, specific and realistic objective, e.g. to be able go shopping.
3. The chosen objective is broken down into small tasks. You may want to use the hierarchy of objectives (see item G and Appendix). Describe each individual task and how it is best accomplished.
4. Describe together different ways in which the objective may be reached (brainstorming). It is important at this stage not to exclude any possible solutions.
5. Weigh the pros and cons of every possible solution. Choose the model that seems the best. It is important that the patient makes the choice.
6. Break down the problem-solving model into steps that are individually manageable. Each task must be clarified in terms of method, time frame and starting point, e.g. the patient may start the first week by taking the dog for a short walk.
7. It may help the patient much if you try to anticipate what will happen and discuss with the patient on beforehand any obstacles that could prevent the plan from being followed.
8. The patient should summarise the problem-solving program and this agenda could have the form of a kind of contract.

The patient will often find the method difficult initially, and it is not unusual that the patient comes to the first sessions without having attempted to use the problem-solving techniques as agreed upon. You should not see this as a problem and do not blame the patient. From a therapeutic point of view, this represents a good opportunity for gaining insight into the patient's understanding of the problem – why is it that the patient has not done as agreed? If it is, for example, due to lack of time, this could indicate that the patient does not take him/herself or the disorder seriously! Instead, you may talk about what was difficult, and what prevented the patient from moving forward.

Basic concepts in cognitive therapy

It is a basic principle of cognitive behavioural therapy that the treatment is targeted, structured and of limited duration. This applies both to individual therapy sessions and the entire therapy. Cognitive behavioural therapy assumes that thoughts and ideas are linked with emotions and actions. Both thoughts and actions can be influenced actively and they will therefore impact emotions and physical reactions, including symptoms. Working with thoughts and ideas allows us to change emotions and actions, and, inversely, behavioural experiments may lead to changes in thoughts, perceptions and emotions.

Psychoeducation, i.e. to teach the patient about the illness and treatment, is an important component of cognitive behavioural therapy. The idea is that the patient learns a way to help him/herself in similar situations – you may say that the patient becomes his/her own therapist. There are a few basic concepts that are central to the cognitive therapy [190]:

+ *Schemata*: General basic assumptions about the person him/herself, others and the world, e.g.: "I must be able to cope with everything".
+ *Basic assumptions/rules of conduct* e.g. "If I can't cope with everything, I'm not worth anything".
+ *Dysfunctional assumptions*: Beliefs about oneself, illness, etc., which may be quite understandable in light of the patient's background (i.e. schemata, basic assumptions and factual knowledge), but which are inappropriate, i.e. they involve medically seen inappropriate illness behaviour, problems with *compliance* in therapy and problems in other ways, thereby preventing the patient from becoming better, e.g.: "If I don't rest, I become more ill".
+ *Automatic thoughts*: Thoughts that arise spontaneously, quickly and often transiently in response to certain impressions and under the influence of underlying schemata and basic assumptions, for example: "I have cancer, I'll die" or "Everyone hates me". Automatic thoughts occur in a given situation and depend to a greater or lesser degree on a *distortion* of this situation made to align it with one's schemata and basic assumptions.
+ *Alternative thoughts*: Other (than the automatic thoughts) possible thoughts in response to an event, e.g.: "Nobody can do everything. Although there are things I cannot do, I am still very valuable", "It's probably a cold and not cancer".

The basic model for cognitive functional disorders
Modification of dysfunctional assumptions and actions

It is important and imperative that the therapy has a specific situation as its point of departure. It may be difficult, especially for a patient with a functional disorder, to identify such a situation, but to help, you may let the patient register symptoms in a table on a weekly basis (Appendix 1). You then choose one episode from the past week. This could be a situation where the symptom was worst, and the GP asks the patient to elaborate the situation.

The Basic Model 1 is completed (Appendix 4A) and you start with the symptoms. If information about emotions, actions, etc. is given, this may be entered along the way. Then you identify automatic thoughts associated with symptoms/illness in the actual episode, for example: "I'll die" or "Now there is a problem with the heart again". If the patient does not continue spontaneously, you may ask what the patient felt about these thoughts and the situation. Again, it should be emphasised that it is important to uncover the spontaneous emotions and not any subsequent rationalisations, e.g. "So you become sad". Then you raise the issue of any actions taken by asking: "What did you do", "How did you handle this", and you may perhaps also ask whether the physical symptoms got better or worse. It is more important that you have a simple and easily understandable example than getting all the details or more examples. The purpose of this method is to make the patient aware of the connection between symptoms, thoughts, emotions and actions and the fact that we cannot directly change physical symptoms or emotions – they are something that we have, but we can change our thoughts and behaviour. There is, so to speak, two handles, you may pull and thus indirectly change the troublesome physical symptoms and emotions.

The next step is to work with alternative thoughts. Basic Model 1 is put aside, but the physical symptoms are carried over to the next step. A brainstorming session with the patient is scheduled where you identify possible and impossible alternative thoughts that the symptoms could have caused. It is important that responsibility for raising creative ideas lies with the patient, but the GP may want to facilitate the process with his own proposals and in some cases also introduce them, even if the patient does not think they are relevant. You should then try to get the patient to make the mental experiment that the alternative ideas were actually true – what feelings would this give rise to in that situation? What actions would this bring and what would the possible consequences be in terms of physical symptoms?

By comparing the feelings and symptoms evoked by alternative thoughts and actions taken in response to these thoughts with those the patient noted in the original basic model, the patient will often experience a whole new world, which brings hope that things might change by using this method of treatment.

Dysfunctional illness beliefs

The patient's own illness beliefs are often of paramount importance for treatment (see TERM Model step A.6 and in Chapter 8 on "Symptom perception"). A dysfunctional illness understanding may hinder treatment if you are unaware of its existence. If the patient, for example, thinks that exercise exacerbates his illness, he will, of course, resist suggestions about physical exercise. In many cases, it takes time to change the patient's dysfunctional illness beliefs. You may yourself contemplate the idea that it has been proved that acupuncture can cure appendicitis. What will it take and how long will it take to convince you of this? Your first instinct will be, never! But please try to think creatively about this possibility. This resembles the task of changing the patient's illness perception, and it is therefore understandable that it takes time to change anything that fundamental. You should thus continue in an empathetic way to work with the patient's illness perception and consequent behaviour as described in step C of the TERM Model. The prerequisite for being able to work with the patient's illness beliefs and illness behaviour is that you know it; it may therefore be necessary to elaborate and further clarify the information that emerged while taking the patient's medical history. If you want to work more intensively with dysfunctional illness perceptions, you may use the form "Cause of Disorder and Symptoms" (Appendix 5). Using dialogue, you may then attempt to get the patient to describe what he/she thought could be the cause of his/her illness/symptoms. It is important to obtain all the explanations, also the unlikely ones. The GP may also make suggestions if relevant. You may then try together with the patient to weigh the pros and cons of every possible causal explanation and, again, it is important that the GP avoids taking the word and leaves it to the patient him/herself to present the arguments – in a dialogue with the GP. Finally, you may talk about the consequences each causal explanation would have, and, possibly, whether and how any possible doubts can be settled. The importance of having a dialogue at this stage of the process and of respecting the patient's thoughts cannot be stressed enough.

Some patients will face difficulties with this technique of weighing for and against, since it is one of the very core problems in this disorder – i.e. that you focus exclusively on a single explanatory model and find it difficult to adopt a broader view. You should therefore not be too persevering and put pressure on the patient, but perhaps just indicate what you know about the problem because you are a medical expert.

Coping – provoking and relieving factors

It is often difficult for patients to identify factors that influence their symptoms. In the aftermath of treatment, it may therefore be necessary to continue the exploration of symptoms. Provoking and relieving factors may, for example, be explored through a diary or a weekly symptom chart (Appendix 1). The result of this exploration is used directly in the cooperation between the patient and the GP to formulate strategies the patient may use to manage his symptoms and problems (coping):

- In the patient's experience, what aggravates his condition?
- What causes symptoms to wear off?
- How has onset of symptoms affected the patient's ability to function?
- How can the patient manage in spite of the symptoms (coping)?

Graded exercise therapy and activation

Where a patient's ability to function is reduced due to functional symptoms, rehabilitation in the form of a gradual increase in activity should be planned [164] (see "Supplementary materials". It is important to be empathic with the patient's fear of the tasks and explain that it will do with steps that are sufficiently small to make the next step manageable. The patient will often become overly optimistic when he begins to feel well again or has a good day, and he will overtax himself and run the risk of being totally exhausted for several days. Such a boom-and-bust behaviour is frequently seen in the most severely ill patients. For example, one day when a patient with a low functional ability was suddenly asymptomatic, she began to roller skate all day and greatly enjoyed being healthy. The following days she had to stay in bed with fatigue, muscle pain, concentration difficulties and many other symptoms. The patient may incorrectly come to the conclusion that physical activity is something that can harm her body. The defeat patients suffer because of this boom-and-bust behaviour could make them lose confidence that treatment options do exist. It is not just physical exercise that may exhaust the patients; also other activities such as socialising and reading may lead to subsequent worsening of their symptoms when the activity becomes exaggerated.

It is therefore important that the challenges are graded and planned so that the challenges, which the patient can safely manage, are tested first. You should gradually proceed from easy tasks to more difficult ones ending with the most severe problems. For this purpose, you may use the staircase form, as discussed in section G "Steps of objectives and list of objectives" (see also Appendices 6 and 7). Moreover, it is important to strike a balance between sufficient activity to continue improvement and not to exaggerate the activity. As a rule of thumb, the patient should physically recuperate so that he/she is able to also exercise the following day. Figure 13.1 may be used to explain to the patient the correct level of training.

Human beings have comfort zones. In that zone, you are relaxed and at a standstill, i.e. in this zone, there is no change or development. Beyond this zone lies a zone where you are challenged. This is where development happens. The outermost zone is one where you are challenged so much that the challenge in itself overtaxes you. If you are constantly living within this outermost zone, you will experience degradation and destruction. The challenge for the patient with a functional disorder is to implement gradual rehabilitation within the zone where there is challenge. The patient must therefore be challenged as much as possible to allow development to take place. But the patient must not be challenged so much that the challenge overtaxes him.

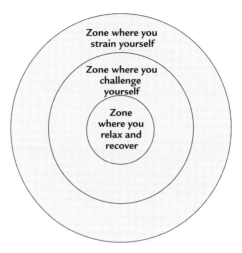

Figure 13.1 Zones of activity (Comfort, challenge, strain)

Steps of objectives and list of goals

It is a basic principle of cognitive behavioural therapy that it should define specific and realistic goals – both the long-term goals of therapy and milestones for each therapy session. The patients' goals are often that they want to become completely well and be like they were before they became ill. This is understandable, but such a goal often seems immense and entirely unattainable for the patient in his/her current state and he/she may therefore despair. Broadly formulated and diffuse goals are difficult to work with in therapy and must be concretised and broken down into a hierarchy of small, manageable operational steps.

You may use the staircase form (Appendix 6) to illustrate this to the patient. Together with the patient, you should set some concrete and realistic goals. The first step is the most important, and it is imperative to set the goals low enough to secure that the patient is successful in reaching the goal and can report this at the next appointment. Example: "I would like to be able to exercise", "We agree that until we meet next time, every day you go and fetch the newspaper in the driveway". Some patients do believe that they are unable to do anything at all. Then you must try to go through their everyday lives – everybody can do something! You may take your point of departure in what the patient is already doing, and then add a little more. You should be aware of any dysfunctional beliefs the patient may have because they may pose a problem to a gradual activation. If the patient, for example, believes that the body will be damaged by the activity, it is clear that he/she will be reluctant to do the activity. This attitude often reflects a distinct black-and-white thinking: "If there is one thing I cannot do, I cannot do anything", and you should try to work on getting the greys out.

Other patients will be inclined to try to do more than what has been agreed, and it is important to point it out if the patient exhibits a boom-and-bust behaviour. The important thing is stability and that the patient learns to respect his/her own limitations, but also to keep on even though it may be difficult at times. It is also important that the patient learns that it does no harm to the body to increase activity and exercise, i.e. if he does not exceed his limits to any extreme degree.

You may also use the list of objectives (Appendix 7) to clarify and identify specific areas that you want to work with. The goals should primarily be formulated by the patient him/herself, but in a dialogue with the GP, who can also contribute with good ideas.

CHAPTER 14

Example of a course of conversations in primary care

LENE TOSCANO AND MARIANNE ROSENDAL

Most general practitioners will be able to have, for example, seven 30-minute conversation sessions with a patient. This chapter outlines how such a course may be planned for a patient with functional symptoms.

Background

A 45-year-old woman who works as a school teacher got divorced 2 years ago and has two boys at home, 14 and 17 years respectively. The woman has been registered with the practice for 15 years. The medical records show that she has not previously had any serious physical disease. She has consulted the practice 4-5 times a year, where she comes to "get checked", typically due to infections or sore muscles. She has been referred to physiotherapy twice because of infiltrations in her back and neck. She has always attended preventive examinations and the children's vaccination programmes. In connection with her divorce 2 years ago, she was ill twice, for 2 and 3 weeks respectively. She had two conversational sessions with the general practitioner in whose records she was described as having a tendency to cry and be confused. It is not clear from the records how she managed to pull herself up again, but she is now working full time. One year ago, the woman had a "health check", where everything was found to be normal.

The woman now consults her general practitioner with various symptoms. Over the past 6 months, she has felt ever more troubled by the pain in her back and neck from which she has been suffering for several years. They tend to disappear when she goes to bed and takes over-the-counter pain killers. Now the pain has grown worse instead, and she sleeps poorly at night, which causes severe fatigue and she has difficulty concentrating. One and a half month ago, a colleague accidentally opened a closet door so that it hit the patient in her head. Since then she has been dizzy, nauseous and has had headaches.

Four weeks ago while shopping, she became so dizzy that she fell on the floor in a supermarket. She struck her right hip, got a very severe headache and her heart was beating so hard and fast that she also had a sore chest. She could not even stand up, and an ambulance was called taking her to the emergency ward. The woman was hospitalised for 2 days and was thoroughly examined for neurological, heart and orthopaedic problems, but nothing pathological was found. During her hospitalisation, a rather unpleasant consultant suggested that it was just "something mental" and that she had had an attack of "hysteria". She was discharged with the message that nothing was wrong.

Since her hospitalisation, the patient has become increasingly poor, she has been forced to take sick leave several times and she is starting to get worried that something is seriously wrong. At work, some colleagues suggested that they think she is off sick too often. One suggested that she should just "pull herself together".

The first regular consultation

The woman now asks her general practitioner to be tested for "everything". She even suspects that she may have a metabolic disorder and fears that she has a tumour in her abdomen. The general practitioner uses a part of the session to make a thorough medical history that ends with a physical examination where blood samples are drawn and the patient is referred to outpatient abdominal ultrasound indicated by a possible filling under the right curvature. Before the patient leaves the clinic, the outcome of the consultation and the examination is briefly summarised. A new session is scheduled for the patient to get the result of the tests.

The second regular consultation

The patient gets the results of the tests and examinations. Everything is normal. She is very frustrated that nobody can figure out what is wrong with her. She has been unable to go to work for 2 weeks and they've phoned from her workplace and asked when she expects to be back. She tells the general practitioner how she now feels. She is having headaches, cannot concentrate, feels as if she is locked in a bell jar, becomes completely exhausted just by walking up the stairs and cannot exercise anymore. She goes to the toilet five times a day and has weird mushy stools, feels constantly bloated and gets stomach cramps that are so severe that she must bend over and sit down. Her heart beats wildly and it can beat so hard that she cannot fall asleep. She has a tingling sensation in her fingers, and she thinks that she shakes and trembles; sometimes it is so violent that others can see it. She ends by saying: "I know nobody else with so many things wrong, who is not ill".

The general practitioner writes down all the patient's symptoms and comes to the conclusion that the patient meets the criteria for having a functional disorder and that she also has been thoroughly examined for any physical disease.

He begins by asking her when the symptoms started, when they are at their worst, and how she otherwise is. It soon becomes apparent that she is extremely overloaded at work and at home, and that there may be a correlation between the extra stress and the exacerbation of her symptoms. They make an appointment for a first of a series of talks.

1st conversation

The session takes the form of a dialogue. It turns out that the patient has a *dysfunctional illness understanding*, where she still believes that her illness has to do with her metabolism. She also thinks that a disease is either "physical" or "mental". She says that her mother had "bad nerves" and that as a child she already decided that she would never end up like her mother. The general practitioner and the patient gradually arrive at a new illness understanding in which she tries to see her symptoms within in a larger bio-psycho-social context. The general practitioner explains to the patient about functional disorders and *bodily distress syndrome*. The GP introduces the weekly symptom chart and asks her to fill it out and bring it to the next consultation.

2nd conversation

The practitioner and the patient go over the weekly symptom chart together. It turns out that she has had 3 episodes of severe exacerbation of symptoms. The 3 episodes were:

1. Severe headaches, blurred vision, palpitations and feeling of numbness in her hands. The symptoms occurred approx. 30 minutes after a colleague had phoned and asked how she felt.
2. Palpitations, dry mouth, shortness of breath, headaches and feeling that the throat shrinks. The symptoms occurred after a conflict with her eldest son who would not accept that he had to be home no later than 10pm on a weekday evening.
3. Headaches, strong fatigue and stomach ache. The symptoms occurred approx. 1 hour after a phone conversation with her ex-husband who asked if he could take his sons on a fishing trip this weekend, although it was planned that the sons would be with her.

All episodes meant that the woman took painkillers (Paracetamol + Ibuprofen) and went to bed.

The session takes the form of a negotiation in which the general practitioner and the patient explore whether there may be a correlation between symptom exacerbations and preceding events. The patient is immediately dismissive of the idea, saying at one point to the general practitioner: "So what you're saying is that this is just something mental?". The general practitioner applies *rope-a-dope*. He listens to her reluctance and agrees that many believe that the symptoms she has are rooted in mental problems and that he can understand why this seems strange given the many physical symptoms. He explains, however, that there are no medical or surgical treatments, and therefore it is important to look at other options. We know that stress can also make you feel physically worse. It is agreed that at the next consultation, the focus will be on the thoughts, emotions and actions that arise in situations where the patient feels she gets worse.

3rd conversation

The patient says that she has been contacted by the school principal, who would like to know when she expects to get back to work. He asked a lot about her illness and insisted that she come to the school for an interview about her illness. Subsequently, she became so ill that she had to stay in bed all day and most of the next day too.

Together the patient and the general practitioner fill in "The cognitive basic model for functional disorders" (found in Appendices 4A and B) with the patient's automatic thoughts and actions (Figure 14.1). The patient and

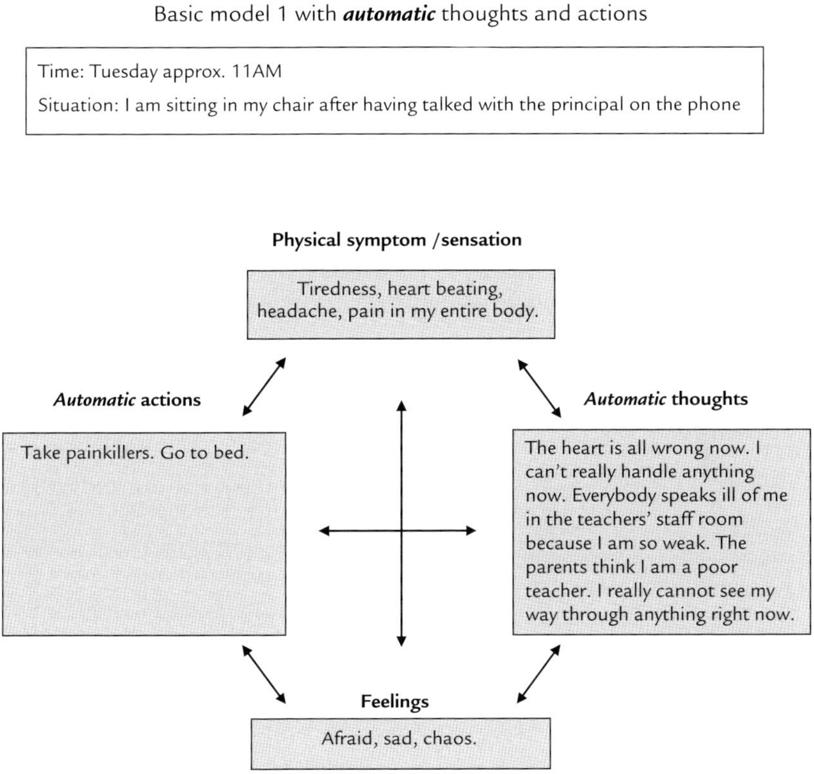

Basic model 1 with *automatic* thoughts and actions

Time: Tuesday approx. 11AM
Situation: I am sitting in my chair after having talked with the principal on the phone

Physical symptom /sensation

Tiredness, heart beating, headache, pain in my entire body.

Automatic actions

Take painkillers. Go to bed.

Automatic thoughts

The heart is all wrong now. I can't really handle anything now. Everybody speaks ill of me in the teachers' staff room because I am so weak. The parents think I am a poor teacher. I really cannot see my way through anything right now.

Feelings

Afraid, sad, chaos.

Figure 14.1 Example of automatic thoughts and actions. See Appendix 4 A for the model.

Basic model 2 with *alternative* thoughts or actions

Time: Tuesday approx. 11AM

Situation: I am sitting in my chair after having talked with the principal on the phone

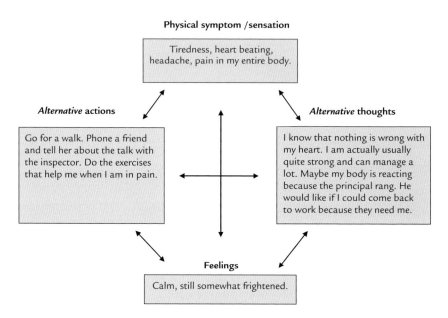

Figure 14.2 Example of alternative thoughts and actions. See Appendix 4 for the model.

the general practitioner work through the possible alternative thoughts (Figure 14.2). It is agreed that the patient completes the basic model when he/she registers a worsening of symptoms and brings it along at the next session.

4th conversation

The patient found working with the basic model rewarding. Several times she found that the alternative thoughts diminished her symptoms. "It is as if the alternative thoughts can bring the whole system to calm down", she says. The general practitioner and the patient go over the charts and the pattern emerges that she often gets symptoms when others expect something from her that she feels she cannot give. Together they find out that she has a basic *schemata*, which can be expressed as follows: "I am a person who is always helping others".

Together, they formulate her *basic assumptions /norms* as follows: "If I do not help others, nobody will like me". The *dysfunctional assumptions*: "If I'm not on top of everything, it is best that I stick to myself, so that I'm not a burden to others". The *automatic thoughts*: "I'm all alone in the world. Nobody likes me".

5th conversation

The patient tells that she has seen a noticeable change in her symptoms. She has been interviewed at work, and she had many symptoms when she came to the school. But she could feel the symptoms wore off when she became aware of the automatic thoughts and had formulated some alternative thoughts for herself. She had great support from the inspector, and they agreed that she should not return to work until she was ready and that she would be able to return at the pace she thought she can handle.

The conversation may be used to review what went well and to dwell upon the successful experience.

6th conversation

The patient has had a good start using the basic model in many situations. But there have been a few episodes of conflict, especially with the eldest son where she cannot find alternative thoughts. It turns out that there were problems with that son a year ago because he was in a group that smoked hash. Back then, a mother from her son's class rang the patient and claimed that her son had been lured into smoking hash by the patient's son.

This was very upsetting to the patient, and it did not help that her son was in the 9th grade at the school where she was employed. She felt that the other teachers frowned on her and thought she was a poor mother. Every time her son was going to a party or going out with friends, she feared that he had started smoking hash again.

Together the patient and general practitioner devised the alternative thought: "Nobody can be the perfect mother. I've done it as best I could. I'll have to trust my son".

7th conversation

The patient tells that the alternative thoughts do not work in her relationship with her son. "I simply cannot accept that I may not be the perfect mum", she says. But she has felt an improvement in many of her symptoms. The symptoms are still there, but not to the same extent as before, and she has become better at finding alternative actions instead of taking medication and going to bed. She thinks that she is now so well that she is ready to work again. It is agreed that she may gradually return to work.

The general practitioner explains and provides the steps of objectives (Appendix 6). The patient finds that it makes good sense and agrees to escalate the amount of work step by step. The objective must be to work 30 hours per week and accept that all tasks cannot always be solved perfectly. She believes that she can continue to work with in steps of objectives and the basic model.

The conversation sessions are terminated, but it is agreed to schedule a general consultation after 6 weeks to discuss the progress made. Moreover, it is stressed that the patient may, of course, contact her general practitioner before this if needed.

PART IV

CHILDREN

CHAPTER 15

Children

CHARLOTTE RASK

Introduction

Special factors in children

- The developmental perspective is essential. The manifestation of a functional physical symptom depends on the child's current stage of development. The types and patterns of symptoms in childhood are therefore different from those reported in adulthood, although there is some overlap. *Example:* There seems to be a link, determined by the developmental course, between problems of regulation in infancy (eating and sleeping problems), functional abdominal pain in childhood and irritable bowel syndrome in adulthood [192;193].
- The linguistic and cognitive development, especially within the first 10 years of life, means that family and other social networks should be involved in the diagnostic assessment.
- In children, family characteristics are particularly important in symptom management, contacts with the healthcare system, health care utilisation, and lifestyle changes. There is often a need for family-based intervention and treatment. *Example:* Both children with chronic fatigue syndrome and functional abdominal pain have a worse prognosis if their parents are convinced that the symptoms can solely be explained by biological factors and/or a physical disease [194-196].

Frequency

Knowledge about the frequency of specific somatoform disorders in children is scarce, but functional symptoms, especially in the form of recurrent pain complaints, are common. In school age, about 1 in 10 children complain about recurring bothersome physical symptoms [197]. Studies on pre-school children are few. A study on 5-7-year-old Danish children found that the 1-year prevalence of parent-reported functional symptoms affecting the child's functional capacity is 4.4% [198]. In older children, like in adults, the prevalence is higher in girls than boys. We have no figures of how many children with functional symptoms are seen in primary care in Denmark. A previous UK study among general practitioners found that psychosomatic-like symptoms were the reason for encounter in 17% of child patients [199]. However, it is certainly not all cases that are seen in primary care. A recent Australian study showed that 44% of the children seen in primary care had had parent-reported abdominal pain during the past year, but in 66% of the cases, the parents themselves handled the symptom without seeing a GP [200]. In the aforementioned Danish study on 5-7-year-olds, 31% of the children with functional symptoms had been in contact with a GP during the past year due to these symptoms.

Table 15.1 Functional physical symptoms in children [197;201-206]

- Are often mono- or oligo-symptomatic, but the frequency of multi-symptomatic presentations increases with age and begins to resemble symptom patters in adults.
- Are most often in the form of recurrent pain such as of headache, stomach ache or pain in arms/legs, especially in young children. Chronic fatigue and neurological symptoms like disturbed gait or sensations and non-epileptic seizures are relatively rare, but become more frequent with age.
- May lead to considerable functional impairment with reduced physical activity, absence from school, negative effect on leisure activities, social isolation and heavy consumption of healthcare services.
- Have, like in adults, a high comorbidity with emotional disturbances (anxiety and depression), but also behavioural problems and learning difficulties may be seen.
- May be accompanied by health anxiety. The specific cognitive disturbances as described in health anxiety in adults with compulsive ruminations over serious illness are, however, rarely demonstrated in small children. The child may, instead, be afraid that something will break in the body, or worries may be expressed in the child's behaviour, e.g. it may be very difficult to comfort the child if it has physical symptoms.

Clinical presentation

Like in adults, functional symptoms in children fall within a spectrum of mild, often self-limiting symptoms to conditions with chronic and debilitating symptoms. The presentation in children, however, differs from that in adults in several ways (Table 15.1).

Diagnostic criteria

Functional symptoms in children usually do not meet the ICD-10 criteria for somatoform disorders and are instead usually classified by non-specific symptom diagnoses. However, the on-going work with ICD-11 will likely imply that the classification of severe functional symptoms in children is improved since children with only a few symptoms may meet the diagnostic criteria for bodily distress syndrome if they experience significant functional impairment (see Chapter 4).

Family factors

Considerable evidence now supports the importance of family factors for functional symptoms in children [207]. Functional symptoms and disorders can present with familial clustering, and children often have symptoms similar to those of other family members. Already from the age of 3 to 4 years, children's understanding of illness behaviour is influenced by and shaped especially by the parents' symptom management, illness perception and possible mental problems [204]. Studies have shown a high degree of parental involvement in the child's illness if the children and adolescents have a functional disorder (chronic fatigue syndrome) compared with parents of children with other disorders. Furthermore, there is an association between both functional disorders as well as anxiety and depression in parents and physical symptoms in children [197]; and parental health anxiety may lead the child to have frequent visits to a GP [208].

Other negative life events and stressors in the home, including poor socio-economic conditions, also increase the prevalence of functional symptoms in children. In individual cases, physical and mental abuse may also be at play. Such abuse is, however, a risk factor for mental health problems in general. It is probably the combination of various stressors, mental difficulties, health problems and a tendency to interpret symptoms as being caused by physical disease (physical attribution) and disease-focused behaviour that lies at the root of the increased incidence of functional symptoms/disorders in some families, where children with a fragile mental constitution (timid, sensitive, conscientious) and increased stress sensitivity seem particularly susceptible.

A two-step explanatory model for the development of severe functional abdominal pain has recently been described. This model integrates current knowledge on the interaction of various important factors, including family factors and the child's individual vulnerability [209]. Since there is an overlap between these findings and findings in other types of functional symptoms in children, the model can be regarded as a more general developmental model for functional disorders in children (Appendix 8).

Diagnostic assessment

There is no validated programme for the diagnostic assessment in children. In the current literature, the following is recommended [210-212].

Medical history

A thorough symptom history should be made on the basis of interviews with both child and parents since children, particularly when younger than 9-10 years, have difficulty describing the duration, course and frequency of their symptoms. In cases where there is no good agreement between parental accounts and self-reported symptoms, the GP should determine which information should be weighted most. The GP must inquire into how the child develops and performs in kindergarten or school, and whether the child is often ill and how the symptoms have affected the child's daily life and leisure activities. Other important information that can support the diagnosis is listed in Table 15.2.

Table 15.2 Information indicating that the symptoms are functional [210;211]

- Co-occurrence of likely stressors and the physical symptoms (e.g. bouts of pain when there are problems in school or family conflicts)
- Psychiatric comorbidity (anxiety, depression or other mental disease) in the child
- Previous functional symptoms in the child and/or a familial clustering of functional disorders
- Social or familial symptom aggravation (e.g. that the child achieves particular benefits or avoids things when it has symptoms)
- A symptom model in the family or in the social environment
- The symptom and/or the degree of functional impairment does not match the clinical findings (e.g. protracted, severe abdominal pain after short-lived gastrointestinal infection)
- Response to psychological treatment, suggestion or placebo

NB: None of these criteria are positive criteria as they are also encountered in children with well-defined physical diseases, but any co-occurrence increases the likelihood.

Questionnaire

The medical history may be supplemented by a questionnaire, e.g. a symptom checklist like the Children's Somatization Inventory (CSI sum score 0-140) that can be filled in by parents and children ≥ 8 years [201;213] (Appendix 9). A high score suggesting more frequent/severe positive complaints over the past two weeks can support the diagnosis. It must, however, be stressed that there are no normal reference values for Danish children, and a high score does not exclude physical disease.

Observation

During the consultation, the GP may also obtain a clinical impression of the child and observe parent-child interaction and parental management of their child.

Physical examination

A physical examination that includes a general physical assessment with measurement of height and weight should be performed.

Para-clinical examinations

The need for additional tests depends on the results of the above procedures. Since symptoms of a physical and functional disorder are similar, a basic investigation programme may be needed that could include Hgb, L+D, platelet count, SR/CRP, liver and blood analysis, TSH and urinary sticks.

Additional information

Other additional information, e.g. from kindergarten/school about the child's cognitive and social functioning and/or the collection and review of past medical records may be relevant.

Treatment

The biggest difference in the treatment of children compared with adults is the need for cooperation with and assistance to the family and other parts of the social network, such as kindergarten or school. The younger the child, the more should focus be on supporting parents and the wider network in the proper management of the child's symptoms. Like in adults, treatment may benefit from a *stepped care* approach.

Mild to moderate functional symptoms

Most children with mild to moderate functional symptoms can often be treated only by reassuring the parents and the child using normalisation, "naming", and offering an explanation of the symptoms, e.g. by using a simple, illustrated explanatory model describing how functional symptoms develop and are sustained [211]. It must be emphasised that the symptoms do not necessarily disappear. The child and its parents should be encouraged to focus on normal activities and behaviour to enhance the family's own coping with the symptoms. Successful treatment may be furthered by disseminating information to the kindergarten/school; for example in the form of a short letter about the child's problem and suggestions on how the kindergarten/school may handle situations in which the child experiences symptoms (e.g., the child should have a short break instead of going home).

There may be a need for cooperation with the school to design a specific plan for the gradual resumption of schooling and activities.

Severe functional symptoms

In difficult and complex cases, like when the child is academically or socially at risk due to long-term absence from school or social contacts, it is often necessary to contact an interdisciplinary team like in a paediatric ward. In such cases, treatment elements could include rehabilitation by physiotherapy and psychological techniques [210;212]. In the most severely affected patients, who may have a high degree of psychiatric comorbidity and dysfunctional illness beliefs and illness behaviour, a joint paediatric and child psychiatric effort can be required. Family-based cognitive behavioural therapy has proven effective in several functional disorders among children and adolescents, but due to the lack of research there is as yet no basis for evidence-based guidelines on specific treatments [214]. Similarly, the implementation of systematised models for shared care for these children is not yet widespread in Denmark.

When the parents' illness behaviour complicates recovery

When the parents' illness behaviour seems to be the primary problem, it is particularly important to examine the parents' own perceptions of illness and any possible health anxiety. Recognition of their concern for the child's symptoms and a focus on any fear of physical disease is of crucial importance for the treatment alliance. It is not always possible to achieve a common understanding. Acceptance of the GP's authority (despite any differences in understanding) may here be a sufficient goal, or the ambition may even be just to protect the child against potentially dangerous investigations. There may be a need for informing the municipality as well as for collaboration with paediatric and/or a child and adolescent psychiatric department.

Medicine

SSRI therapy may be indicated in cases with comorbid anxiety and/or depression [210]. Initiation of SSRI treatment of children is a specialist task, while maintenance therapy in consultation with a specialist in child and adolescent psychiatry may be handled by the general practitioner (please refer to the relevant national authority for any guidelines on the treatment of children with psychoactive drugs including antidepressants).

CHAPTER 16

Cultural approaches to the study of functional disorders

TRINE DALSGAARD, ANN OSTENFELD-ROSENTHAL AND METTE BECH RISØR

Symptoms for which an explanation cannot readily be found, combined with frequent visits at the general practitioner and concern for one's own health, are increasingly seen as a phenomenon that we all know and feel to a various degree. Simultaneously, awareness is growing that diseases can rarely be said to be purely biological or psychosocial phenomena, and this realisation dissolves the sharp distinction between the two theoretical concepts of illness and disease. In other words, the approach to functional disorders in anthropology today is characterised by the fact that it is not seen as a discrete disorder; rather, it is increasingly acknowledged that all suffering contains a degree of somatisation and all disease processes challenge the division between body and psyche.

The following chapter summarises some of the changes the cultural approaches to the study of functional disorders have undergone over the past 30 years. These changes reflect developments within general anthropology as well as the societal shift from modernisation to post-modernisation [215]. The modern era, the epoch of the grand narratives, can be said to be characterised by growing differentiation and rationalisation. Today, these processes are becoming ever more dissolved and mixed. Post-modern society thus differs from modern society in that it is characterised by fragmentation followed by a convergence into new constellations and brings into question the pervasiveness of rationality. Still, there is little agreement whether we are in a post-modern era or not. The above does, however, set a scene of upheaval and the creation of new definitions in many fields, e.g. the individual's illness understanding, social development and different scientific paradigms like health sciences and anthropology.

A few anthropologists have addressed somatisation issues in recent years. In Denmark, for example, such researchers include the three authors of the present Part V of this book, but the field has also seen contributions from French, Spanish and, in particular, British researchers. The field has also attracted several sociologists, health psychologists, philosophers, etc. from many countries who follow the same paths as anthropology. The rest of the chapter will review typical ways in which attempts have been made to apply socio-cultural dimensions to the study of somatisation regardless of the research disciplines applied. It is inherently an incredibly broad field, wherefore some writers have been selected to represent typical time trends in the cultural approaches to the study of somatisation. Thus, the review is far from complete, but should be seen as a summary of some dominant trends rooted in anthropology.

Background – anthropology and the body

Somatisation has only relatively recently become a field of research in anthropology, mainly because the subject field of anthropology has undergone a number of drastic changes during history. Modernity was dominated by various scientific directions seeking maximal variation. As far as the study of the human body was concerned, this meant that there was often a sharp division between biological and social explanations. The body was long considered relatively uninteresting in anthropology, because culture was considered to be in the mind and not in the body, reflecting the prevailing dualistic thinking.

When anthropology broadened its focus to include the body, it was initially viewed as a means with which to express culture. Although a critique of this view of the body and a call for a socio-psycho-biological study of the body [216] was voiced already in 1935, the goal of most anthropological studies of the body remained to demonstrate the imperative of culture in matters of bodily expression. The body was thus for many years reduced to a symbol of society, a tabula rasa, a clean slate, on which culture could set its stamp.

The former anthropological view of the body enrolled itself into the dualistic mind/body philosophy and the focus of the debate remained whether bodily expressions were universal and biological or relative and cultural/social. This dualistic approach to the study of the body prevailed, even when anthropology began to see the body as a means of communication in the sense that it was seen mainly as an object of communication, i.e. the body remained a passive object on which culture could set its stamp, or it was a manifestation of thought and hence remained placed in a hierarchical relationship where it was inferior to the mind. Only in the late 1970s did this passive perception of the body begin to change. 1977 saw the release of "Towards an anthropology of the body" [217], where J. Blacking as one of the first anthropologists insisted on the importance of emotions in the study of the body. The body and consciousness were seen not as independent contrasts, and Blacking thereby attempted to overcome "dualism". This approach to the body is phenomenological in the sense that phenomenology, in anthropology, refers to the human experience of being in the world and hence adopting the world in a pre-conscious, bodily way. Methodically, social phenomena are understood from the actors' own perspectives and the approach describes the world as it is experienced by the informants. Basically, the working premise is that reality is what people perceive it to be. However, this phenomenological approach to the body fitted poorly into the prevailing modernist thinking and, with a few exceptions, it only came to influence the study of the body somewhat later.

It is thus no coincidence that somatisation viewed from a more anthropological perspective did not really become a field of study until the mid-seventies, as the body first had to be legitimised as an anthropological object of study by slowly moving away from the dualistic thinking that characterised modernity.

The study of somatisation – a historical perspective
The discussion on culture-bound syndromes (CBS)

The anthropological study of somatisation sprang, inter alia, from the discussion about culture-bound syndromes, i.e. *"A class of abnormal and pathological patterns found in non-western societies which cannot be explained readily in Western psychiatric terms"* [218 p. 5], such as Latah in Malaysia Latah defined by Winzeler as: *"A nervous affection characterised by an exaggerated physical response to being startled or unexpected suggestion, the subject involuntarily uttering cries or executing movements in response to command or imitation of what they hear or see in others ..."*

In the first half of the last century, other races were generally regarded as less intelligent, which characterised the discussion of culture-bound syndromes. The "foreigners" were ascribed traits that presented them as inferior, such as being more anxious than Western people, and they therefore acquired culture-specific diseases. In the second part of the last century, the discussion turned to focus on problematising the concept because it gradually became clear that culture-bound syndromes also existed in the West, which gave a new dimension to the concept. Initially, this consisted of an appreciation of other dimensions of disease than physical errors (see *illness/ disease* discussion below), and, subsequently, several Western diagnoses were problematised as cultural, for example in the discussions about anorexia and bulimia. This meant that the many different symptoms, combined under the term CBS, were increasingly being brought into question, and it was discussed how specific a syndrome should be to be culturally specific and not universal or rather trans-cultural. Medical anthropologists and some sociologists and psychologists began to dissolve the Western diseases for which unique causal explanations (either biological or psychological) had previously been sought, and they showed that they were context-dependent, at least partially. This reflected the rising acceptance of relativism in science generally where people began even to question if health was relative and thus question the existence of universal diagnoses.

It was, among other things, this growing acceptance of the influence of culture, also on Western diagnoses, that paved the way for the study of Western diseases, including that of functional disorders, as relevant objects of anthropological exploration. After this outline of the development of the body and functional disorders as anthropological objects of scientific study, the following section will outline the evolution in the cultural approaches to functional disorders over the past 30 years.

The 70s: Criticism of biomedicine and focus on the illness experience

The anthropological study of somatisation is, in other words, relatively new. The subject began to become popular in the late 70s when Kleinman et al. published the article "Depression, somatization and the new cross-cultural psychiatry" [219]. In line with the previous section, this article was written as an argument against what Kleinman called *the old transcultural psychiatry*, which often ended in a search for universal features transcending cultures because researchers were looking for a basic core of diseases. Kleinman criticised the search for common characteristic disease traits because this very search precluded the identification of culture-specific aspects of the disease. Kleinman explicitly problematised Western diagnoses as culture-bound and described the entire biomedical model as just one of many medical systems. In other words, already here, Kleinman expressed his doubts about the universal nature of illness as something that could be detected in a pure biological form below the cultural layers. Kleinman therefore calls for a more detailed, local and phenomenological study of the forms of expression of suffering and hence continued the prevailing discussion about the relationship between *illness* and *disease* by insisting on the importance of the study of *illness*. *Illness* is defined by Kleinman as "*the way individuals and the members of their social network perceive symptoms, categorize and label those symptoms, experience them, and articulate that illness experience through idioms of distress and pathways of help seeking*". *Disease* is defined as "*the way the illness experience is reinterpreted by practitioners in terms of their theoretical models and through clinical work*" [220 p. 225]. *Illness* and *disease* were seen then as two phenomena that existed independently of each other and therefore basically were two separate study areas, respectively, social and biological. Although Kleinman retains the fundamental distinction between *illness* and *disease* in the article, he begins at the same time to see manifestations of culture in both *illness* and *disease* and to treat *disease* not simply as a purely biomedical reality, but also as socially constructed. Thus, already at that time, a rebellion against the sharp distinction between *illness* and *disease* begins.

To sum up, the study of somatization in anthropology began mostly as a critique of the medicocentrism and ethnocentrism of biomedicine with criticism of biomedicine for its lack of understanding of patients' life-worlds and its universalist approach to disease diagnoses, which was the basis for comparative studies. The concept of ethnocentrism refers to the use of one's own society as a benchmark for other communities which makes them appear inferior. This concept has been transferred to biomedicine as "medico-centrism" which refers to a critique of the way in which biomedicine looks at illness categories in other societies. Bordering on this concept is "medicalisation", which, however, signifies the extent to which every conceivable phenomenon in our own society is subsumed under the biomedical domain and viewed as disease and health [221].

The first real cultural studies of somatisation behaviour were part of this discussion and therefore focused on *illness*, i.e. the personal experience of disease. Often this approach was accompanied by ignorance of how the concept of *disease* and other external factors dynamically influenced the *illness* experience. In other words, it is easy to indulge into studying *illness* without taking into account that *illness* and *disease* are two sides of the same coin and that they are an analytic phenomena, artificially separated for the sake of analysis, but, for example, do not exist as separate empirical forms. Any patient always has (at least) both an *illness* experience and a *disease* understanding of a disease, and so has a health professional for that matter. Analytically, you may choose to weigh one over the other, but the balance often ends as a reductionist approach. On the other hand, the priority given to *illness* is an attempt to promote the illness perspective of a disorder, where approaches in other perspectives have mainly been *disease*-dominated.

Kleinman was definitely the leading figure in the study of the cultural aspect of the functional disorders in the seventies. He describes his development in a later interview: "[...] *I became much more aware of the [...] importance of just seeing things in terms of the local world of patients and practitioners [...] In the seventies I moved from a cognitive orientation, with the social and the cognitive together, into increasingly an orientation around experience...*" [222 p. 112]. The *illness* experience thus remained the focus of many studies during the eighties.

The 80s: Further development

The discussion about the relationship between *illness* and *disease* was gradually deepened in the early 80s owing, among others, to Ford, who explicitly addresses their dialectical relationship. *"All disease processes appear to be influenced by psychosocial stressors, and, in a reciprocal fashion, the psychological state of the patient is influenced by the disease"* [82 p. 5]. The distinction between *illness* and *disease* thus began slowly to dissolve, since more researchers began to question whether a disease could be understood using a biomedical approach only. At the same time, however, the body was still often seen as an object managed by the psyche (consciously or unconsciously). Focus was often on somatising people as a separate population group with problems of expressing feelings verbally, or somatisation was seen as a way of communicating to and controlling the local environment. These views left little space for the cultural dimension and did not include how socio-culture manifests itself in the event. *Disease* and *illness*, in other words, remain in the body.

The breakdown of disorders into *illness* and *disease* has thus occupied a central position in cultural approaches to somatisation. This division has characterised much of the discussion, especially in the 80s, which should also be seen in light of the fact that the body in some way still had not gained a status as a legitimate object of anthropological study. Yet, in its ambition to achieve legitimacy, anthropology helped maintain a dualistic way of thinking about the body because culture was all too often considered to be crucial. This made anthropology open to the same criticism as that which had been directed against others, namely that anthropologists fell victims of reductionist thinking, whether it was psychological reductionism or bio-reductionism. This was reflected in the modernist mind-set in the sense that it was characteristic that the professions "totalised" their respective perspectives and thus excluded other professional perspectives. In other words, the study was characterised by the belief that disorders could be explained by simple causal factors and that there was a truth, whether it was biological or psychological or, in this case, cultural.

Already in 1980, Kleinmann commented on some of the problems that arose by splitting *illness* and *disease* into two concepts and thus continued, among other things, the process that had begun in 1977, namely Blacking's move towards a more phenomenological approach to man in the world. The division into *illness* and *disease* was beginning generally to be called into question because these fields were considered simplistic and overlapping, and this controversy further gave rise to doubts about whether a disorder was located in the psyche or in biology; a debate that gained momentum again 10 years later both within anthropology and health science.

Most anthropological approaches to the study of somatisation during the 80s were marked by a division in which culture was reduced to something external and no focus was given to the dynamic interplay between individual, body and culture. This was also the case in the late 80s, even if ever greater attention was being paid to the impact of societal discourses on how people perceived and expressed disorders. This is evident also in historical overviews of changes in somatisation phenomenon over time.

But at the same time as a more critical view of society's impact on disorders evolved, the 'culture of disorder' was conceived as something entirely social, i.e. culture or society were, again, not perceived as being in a dynamic interaction with or actively impacting the body. The body and its expression were seen as a result of other external influences, which dictated the form of suffering. The body was therefore even here seen as a symbol of the underlying culture and society, though not always to the same passive extent as in the past. Especially in the late 1980s, the body was given a more active role and was seen as more than a passive object to be fitted into the culture, and illness begins increasingly to be interpreted as *"a form of communication – the language of the organs– through which nature, society and culture speak simultaneously"* [192 p. 183].

Sociosomatics

Even if it is not possible to set fixed dates at which new ways of thinking about particular concepts emerged, Kleinman's introduction of the concept sociosomatics marks a drastic change. In "Social Origins of Disease and Distress" [220], Kleinman speaks about the social influences on cognition, emotions and physiology. According to Kleinman, individuals are connected by a *sociosomatic reticular* which refers to both a bond between individuals and between individuals, and the local system in which they are living. The individual is thus positioned in a social and cultural network or a context that cannot be separated from the individual. The distinction between the physical and social/cultural human thus becomes an analytic construction because the individual as he/she exists and lives cannot be separated from the surroundings. Physical symptoms thus have a social and not only a psychological or biological origin. Kleinman begins to interpret somatisation explicitly as an expression of interpersonal/social suffering, a kind of cultural experience with roots in the political and social structures and processes as well as in the clinical picture. Kleinman tries to link the societal, cultural and individual levels, *illness* and *disease*, and thus to move away from the dualistic thinking. Consequently, he increasingly looks at somatisation as a regular universal phenomenon, where "the body mediates between the social world and the inner world, and, therefore, becomes a means of both representing and expressing, in a more metaphorically sophisticated sense, not just the clinical, but the social problems" [222 p. 113].

This reinforces the criticism of the dominant biomedical model of disease, since it only searches for the origin of disease within the body. This development is also gaining momentum within the medical profession. Somatisation is sought normalised and generalised by connecting the cultural and the individual dimensions. "*Therapists must learn to read the idiom of the body both as a unique metaphoric production of the patient and as a culturally prescribed code that the individual utilizes at times without fully comprehending its wider implications*" [224 p. 13]. The general awareness of the social body is heightened and a gradual dissolution of the boundaries between the social and the individual levels begins: "[…] *what matters in the space of the moral crosses over into what matters in emotions and the space of the body*" [222 p. 118].

Despite these efforts, much of the anthropological literature from the 80s remained focused on the individual's personal experience and the rationale of the individual's behaviour. That is, the main focus was on *illness* experience, studied for instance through narratives or other situational and contextual analyses where the problem area was the subjective experience only. Thus, the anthropological study of functional disorders continued for some time as a critique of the biomedical approach to patients by insisting on the opposite, equally reductionist position.

The 90s: Embodiment and context

"It's getting harder and harder to talk about it [medical anthropology] as a field because there are so many sub-fields in it that I am not sure how the whole relates to the parts [...] There was a time when the field was small enough that I really felt I had an understanding of what was going on. Now it is so large that such a general understanding is impossible" (Kleinman [222, pp. 121-3]. Medical anthropology begins to expand in line with societal changes, and many different trends in the cultural study of functional disorders emerge during the 90s.

The early 90s were characterised by a focus on the broad socio-cultural processes; however, they were still often referred to as unique in their influences on matters relating to the body. For example, much emphasis was given to the shown correlation between socioeconomic factors and disease, but the understanding of this context and the processes that were involved remained negligent. The general movement continues, however, away from reductionist theories towards holistic thinking that acknowledges the interaction between circumstances.

By extension, the functional somatic symptoms were increasingly interpreted not as an expression of a fundamental and categorical diagnosis, but more as a general human response to various issues. This is reflected, for example, in Kleinman's studies that continue to replace the entire concept of psychosomatics with sociosomatics – i.e. a constructed, contextual, historical process that inscribes the social and cultural world of the body. The focus is here increasingly on the collective consciousness embedded in individuals, and you may speak of local/cultural biology [225] where the individual's body is influenced by social and cultural factors that are beyond the individual's reach. This is very unlike the "classic" psychosomatic idea which implies a naturalistic conception of the body as an alternative representation of individual psychological difficulties.

The focus in the 80s on patients' subjective narratives also meant that disease classifications became ever more eroded as patients' subjective narratives hampered the claim to classificatory boundaries because these narratives did not fall into any single categories. Focus thus shifted to a re-classification of the functional somatic disorders, and it was proposed already in the early 90s to focus more on the similarities between the different somatisation diagnoses than to classify them in isolation. In this way, functional disorders came to be seen increasingly as a reflection of the socio-cultural currents since the core basis of suffering was dissolved and increasingly replaced with the idea of *languages of suffering* [226]. This implies that the expression of all medical disorders is seen as a kind of language shaped by cultural patterns and discourses – i.e. the form that symptoms and behaviours take is basically tied to culture. This is seen for example in the experiences of and responses to pain, which are not only physically and personally conditioned, but reflect cultural discourses, i.e. in the sense that they express how it is acceptable and legitimate to express pain [220;226]. The dualistic and classificatory thinking that formerly characterised the study of the functional disorders thus becomes increasingly challenged in the 1990s.

At the same time, focus is retained on the individual body, but now as a living body, i.e. a phenomenological approach is taken where you just recognise that the body and one's reactions are not static, but change with the context. The focus is thus on the experience in context (as opposed to the body), i.e. the interpersonal and individual dimensions are linked. The awareness grows that disorders are social processes, i.e. focus shifts to how disease culture is affected by cultural expectations and the specific social context – for example, power, politics, human relations, morality, poverty, isolation, stigma, etc. Thus, it is increasingly stressed that the illness experience and hence the disease culture is shaped as much by the intersubjective as the individual dimension.

Within these frameworks, the ambition of anthropology is to study and analyse the different levels at which culture interacts and communicates, i.e. to relate the personal level to the interpersonal space and the external discourses – spheres that were previously sharply separated. We are working generally towards a reconciliation of the socio-cultural level with the lived life without working squarely within an *illness/disease* model.

In summary, a movement is seen away from the symptom-focused and other core-oriented descriptions towards the social course in illness culture, which, in itself, affords more space to the cultural studies. Acceptance of multi-factorial influences in functional disorders is growing, i.e. the phenomenon is increasingly seen as a conflation of psychological, biological, social, cultural and historical factors. This connection is seeing a shift towards the social and away from the cognitive dimension. In anthropology, focus is thus on the embodiment of socio-cultural trends because we lack knowledge about how societal discourses become natural to the body and make us act and interpret our lived lives in natural ways in relation to social and cultural meanings systems.

Explanations are gradually abandoned that closely link disorder to the Western view of the individual as a finite essence and a movement towards more social explanations is seen. With this, discourses and ideas are seen in which disorders are partially constructed, and the concept of normality is not uniquely linked to the biomedical explanatory model. Today's approach to how we perceive and define phenomena has hence become more reflective. One final central point in this context is that especially over the last few years, this reflexive science has also come to be characterised by the very theorisation about the body, and disorders themselves become the object of social science, i.e. attention is directed towards the production of knowledge and the processes involved. In the Danish context, the last 10 years have, for example, seen more anthropological and qualitative research into functional disorders than ever seen in the past, mainly owing to the creation of the Research Centre for Functional Disorders and Psychosomatics. Part of this research continues to take its starting point in *illness*, e.g. by theoretically seeking to identify narratives, explanatory disease models or patients' relations to and communication with health care professionals [73,227-233]. On top of this, these efforts are continually open to how a functional disorder is shaped by the dynamic aspects of patients' stories and life-worlds, the practical social processes involved in disease behaviour, the identity that springs from having a chronic disease, as well as the context and social developments. This implies that focus is on the nature of the health-understanding in question and how it is produced, how diagnoses are made and conceived outside the clinical world, and how symptoms and explanatory models are produced as a result of politico-economic factors, social relations, etc. At the root of this approach lies an analytical preoccupation with developments in medicine and health sciences where basic knowledge theory, dualism and universality are being ever more intensely discussed and criticised. This trend is also seen outside Denmark, especially in the sociologist Monica Greco's work with psychosomatics and the construction of illness and body in both a political, social and medical context [234-236]. Greco sides with others, for example the sociologist Nettleton

[237;238]. In the United Kingdom, health psychologists and GPs have also contributed with much insight into GPs' and patients' negotiations on diagnoses and disease explanations in primary care – not only from an *illness* perspective, but also with an eye for how legitimacy, power positions and patient roles must necessarily be produced and used strategically in a patient-therapist relationship. This chapter mentions only a single paper, but the research group has published many papers on this topic [239]. France and Spain as well as other Nordic countries than Denmark have seen similar developments within functional disorders – even if most countries have made less progress than Denmark and the UK. Much research is still at a very early stage and still seeking to identify problem areas seen from a patient perspective that patients experience and have to live with, while Denmark and the UK have gone more to the root of the problem and sought to address the issue by adopting a critical, multidimensional approach to both *illness* and *disease*, and to the individual and society.

Because the healthcare system, by its very nature, is facing difficulties in treating patients with functional disorders, some patients have recently turned to alternative methods which, in general, have seen a proliferation. Especially abroad (i.e. in the UK and the US), a number of quantitative, but very few qualitative, studies have explored patients with functional disorders and their use of alternative treatments. The same is true in Denmark. The themes raised in the Danish studies primarily address the meaningfulness of alternative treatment, the therapist-patient relationship, patients' perception of alternative treatment and the placebo effect [229;240]. However, a number of studies of the so-called culture-bound syndromes have also been published among which we will only mention a few, such as *susto* in Latin America [241-243] and *somatization* in Taiwan [244;245].

Summary

It was fairly straightforward to summarise the developments seen in the '70s; but, today, the picture has become more complex since trends are many and diverse as a result of the general transformation of society and science. Still, a brief summary of developments in the cultural approach to the study of somatisation over the past 30 years shows a movement away from the one-sided explanations, i.e. where somatisation is explained either from a cultural or a biomedical perspective, towards explanations that see suffering from multiple, simultaneous and equal perspectives. We have moved away from the more linear explanations where perspectives were prioritised and clear-cut, and cause-and-effect explanations were offered towards a more simultaneous approach. Today's focus is on the specific contexts in which disorders exist without neglecting the larger context or the complexity of the interaction between *disease* and *illness*. In the postmodern perspective, medicine is seen as a part of the historical development, which lies far from the classic modernist idea of disease and health as part of a discrete, individual body. Kleinman summarises this development thus: *"[...] from the medical systems [...] towards the lived experience of suffering, toward medical practice as a historicised mode of social being-in-the-world [...], from symbolic forms and structure, towards subjectivity and then on to intersubjectivity of experience [...] Medical and psychological categories give way to ethnographic interpretation of intersubjectivity"* [246 p. 6].

This broad view of the somatisation phenomenon as just one of several phenomena that manifest as they do because of the socio-cultural trends also implies that somatising behaviour is increasingly considered a tendency that affects everyone. This implies that disorders are rarely considered to be purely biological or psychosocial, which dissolves the sharp distinction between *illness* and *disease*. Today's anthropological approach to functional disorders is thus characterised by the fact that it is no longer seen as a distinct disorder, but increasingly as a part of any human suffering since the physical and cultural body should be considered as an analytic construct. Anthropology is working towards replacing the traditional, unique and classificatory approach to the field with a more multifactorial approach through an integration of the individual, the interpersonal and the discourse levels. The immediate goal of anthropology in the study of the body and somatisation processes is thus to develop new theories and methodological approaches where the individual disease perception is placed not only in a specific social context, but also in a broader cultural context.

CHAPTER 17

Medico-historical background

PER FINK

Providing an overview of the historical background of functional disorders is difficult for several reasons. Firstly, there is terminological confusion in the field [247]. The term hysteria has been in use since ancient times, but broad consensus on the meaning of the term has never been reached. The term hysteria has consequently been omitted entirely from the ICD-10 [247] and from the American psychiatric classification, as well as from the introduction of the DSM-III [249] in the 1980s. Instead, the term *somatoform disorders* was adopted as a general term for a group of mental disorders that predominantly manifested themselves as physical symptoms. The diagnosis of hysteria was renamed *somatisation disorder* (somatisation condition), covering a group of chronic somatising patients with multiple, medically unexplained, physical complaints as well as *conversion disorder* in the ICD-10: dissociative disorders comprising patients who presented pseudo-neurological symptoms, e.g. paresis. Other subgroups of somatoform disorders are hypochondria and somatoform pain.

The most widespread term used in recent decades is somatisation, which originates from psychodynamic theory. The term is used to describe the process whereby emotional tension manifests in physical symptoms. Attempts have later been made to change its meaning to be purely descriptive; a phenomenon where a patient presents with medically unexplained symptoms, i.e. to use the term as a superordinate term stripped of any hypotheses about its underlying mechanisms [250]. The term *somatoform disorders* is not a comprehensive term that covers all aspects embraced by the concept of somatisation, since, for example, diagnoses like neurasthenia or the newer term chronic fatigue syndrome and *disordo factitius* are not included.

The term psychosomatic disorders was used about physical suffering which was believed to be caused by psychological trauma and conflicts (e.g. *arthritis rheumatica* and *asthma bronchiale*). Later, the term was also used about patients who presented with physical symptoms with no organic basis. The term has now largely disappeared from scientific discourse, but it is still commonly used among laypeople and clinicians.

Today, the term medically unexplained symptoms is frequently used as a non-theoretical, purely descriptive term designating a clinical problem. The term has the disadvantage that it excludes that the disorder may have an organic basis.

Another main problem in a historical overview is that various medical specialties and traditions as well as various lines of research and theorising have developed in parallel. This has led to the development of a wide range of diagnostic labels that are strongly overlapping for the same types of patients which have been designated in different ways. This has led to the emergence of a wide range of syndrome diagnoses that have been in vogue for certain periods, only later to be replaced by other names. Contemporary examples include fibromyalgia, irritable bowel syndrome and multiple chemical sensitivity. In Denmark we speak also about the "new diseases", but viewed from a historical perspective, this seems to be an absurd name.

Many of these oddities in our classification system spring from a failure to abide by the fundamental principles in basic clinical epidemiology and nosology and from the practice of making generalisations on the basis of case stories and highly selected, unrepresentative patient populations. With the perspective offered by historical hindsight, many of the scientific deadlocks in which we also find ourselves today in this area become clearly visible, and the perhaps most striking thing is that our fundamental understanding has not changed as radically as we would like to think.

This review will use the term functional disorders as a general term for the entire group of disorders. The term has been used for centuries [251], but won a foothold especially in neurology where it was partly used in a physiological sense, i.e. for disorders where there were functional disturbances but no structural, organic changes; partly in a more psychological sense about dysfunction caused by intellectual or emotional disturbances. In the sense used here, it is a purely descriptive term that does not indicate unproven hypothetical causal relationships, but simply that there is a functional disturbance. One study has shown that patients perceive the term as neutral and non-stigmatising [31].

The earliest known descriptions of hysteria are found on Egyptian papyrus scrolls dated to about 1900 before our time. Since it is the name that has been used for the longest time and that is most common in writings, a historical overview would necessarily focus on the history of hysteria. A more thorough historical review does not fall within the scope of the present book, but reference may be made to a number of monographs and summary articles [28;250-255].

The migrant uterus

Hippocrates (460 BC) is the founder of modern medical science since he introduced the doctrine that diseases are not caused by supernatural forces like possessions and demons, but by natural phenomena. He emphasised the importance of uncovering the causal relationships in a disease because it was the basis for rational treatment, i.e. a treatment directed against the cause of the disease.

Hippocrates' perception of hysteria much resembled the description found in the early Egyptian papyrus scrolls. It was assumed that hysteria was due to a migrant uterus, i.e. a displacement of uterus. For example, respiratory distress and *globus hystericus* (i.e. a lump in the neck) was ascribed to pressure from the uterus which had drifted up into the abdomen, or the neck, respectively. If it settled at the level of the heart, the patient would feel anxiety and constipation. Spells of cramps and other symptoms believed to be connected to hysteria were explained in similar ways. The anatomical nonsense of such drifting seemed to pose no problem to doctors of that time.

It was the doctor's duty to investigate the patient and to locate the drifting uterus, and any treatment undertaken was to prevent further dislocation, e.g. by using a diaphragm or a tight band around the abdomen so that the uterus could not get past. Attempts were also made to entice or scare the uterus back into place. Either by using fragrant substances and fumes dis-

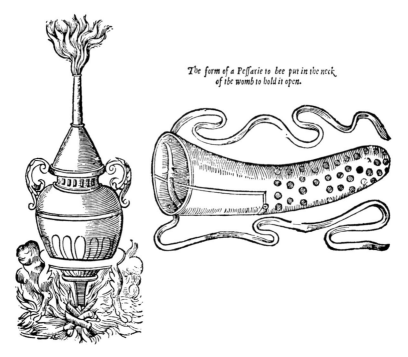

The form of a Pessarie to bee put in the neck of the womb to hold it open.

Figure 17.1 **Parés instruments for the treatment of hysteria [252].** Left: instrument for application of steam into the uterus. Right: a pessary to be injected into the patient's vagina. The holes create the possibility of putting steam into the womb.

pensed into the vagina and/or by using horrid smelling substances/vapours applied in the nose and mouth, or bathing, cold/heat, etc. (see Figure 17.1).

The migration of the uterus was attributed to its drying out and loss of weight because of sexual abstinence. It would therefore migrate towards the hypochondrium and the abdomen to get fluids and air. Treatment therefore encompassed advice that women should marry. Plato even thought that the uterus was an animal who longed to produce children. If it remained infertile for too long after puberty, it became frustrated and drifted around in the body, which continued until the uterus was satisfied by passion and love [252 p. 7].

Seminal retention

Galen (129-199 AD) and others of his contemporaries, Soranus (93-138 AD), contested that the uterus was an animal and that it could migrate, but they did not deny that it was the reason for hysteria and a number of attacks or seizures [252 p. 28]. Galen thought that women produced a secretion in their uterus analogous to the male sperm, and that the cause of hysteria was that this secretion was retained in the uterus due to sexual abstinence, in the same way as menstrual blood could be retained. This *seminal retention* could poison the blood or cool the body which could lead to various sorts of hysterical attacks. Because semen could also be retained in men, they, too, could also get hysterical bouts. Treatment consisted, among other things, in digital manipulation of the uterus to release the secretion. Treatment principles from antiquity are described as late as in a textbook from 1910 by A. Strumpell [28].

Like possession

Christianity became increasingly popular during the 4th and 5th centuries, i.e. after Galen's death, and the Christian Church became the dominant force in society. St. Augustine (354-430 BC) was a very industrious theological writer, and his teachings dominated for the next 1000 years. The church was strongly dogmatic and allowed no innovation, and there was therefore virtually no progress in medical science during this period. With St. Augustine came a return to the old ideas from before Hippocrates, i.e. that evil forces were the cause of all suffering. This view had never lost its grip on the population and is presumably latently present in the population even today, where various healing practices in the form of healing by a touch of the hands, sacred springs, etc., may still be found. St. Augustine believed that all human suffering, including diseases, was due to the fact that the person had been possessed by a devil or another evil force because the person had previously committed a sin [252 p. 49]. He also believed that sex was repulsive and linked to pleasure. Carnal desires were associated with demons and witches, and the sexual act was only legitimate in relation to reproduction.

St. Augustine changed his perception of hysteria from being a disease, which caused both physical as emotional suffering in man to reflect the fact that a human being, more or less against his will, had been obsessed or was in collusion with the devil. Treatment of hysteria was not considered a medical task since it consisted of exorcism, which was a theological responsibility. This meant that in the following centuries, people who suffered from hysteria (as well as other mentally ill patients) were subjected to severe suffering and sometimes torture.

An important proof that a woman was a witch was the finding of an area of the skin that lacked sensibility. Most of the women who were doomed to be witches and burned at the stake in the 16th and 17 century were hysterics, and their "victims" paralysis, blindness, strange behaviour, etc. was probably also manifestations of hysteria [252 p. 61]. The Scottish doctor Jordan in 1603 sought to rescue a young girl from being burned at the stake as a witch by explaining the signs as part of the nature of hysteria [252 p. 120].

Although Galen was not a Christian, he believed in supernatural forces, and he was therefore tolerated by the church fathers. In the absence of novel thinking, his writings acquired almost dogmatic status among the doctors who, despite everything, still practiced throughout the Middle Ages, even if in the hiding.

In the late 16th century, science began to gain foothold again, and the thread from Galen was taken up [252 p. 112]. Hippocrates was rediscovered and his ideas have since had an extraordinary influence on medical science.

Reflex theory

Spinal irritation and the reflex theory were prominent paradigms in medical thinking and practice, especially in connection with hysteria in the latter half of the 19th century. The theories originated in two empirical observations.

In a series of physiological studies in the period 1757-1766, A von Haller from Göttingen showed that a slight stimulation of a muscle produced a disproportionately violent motion reaction – the muscle was very irritated [28 p. 21]. This experiment gave rise to the spinal irritation theory which claimed that all body tissues were irritable or excitable. Diseases occurred either when the tissue was under-excited (*asthenic*) or over-excited (*sthenic*). This condition was generally called inflammation in the presence of objective findings like purulent matter; otherwise, it was called irritation, which covered a wide spectrum of disorders.

In 1750, the Edinburghian doctor R. Whytt demonstrated the existence of reflex arcs the centre of which was the spinal cord (e.g. the knee jerk reflex). The anatomical explanation for reflex arcs, however, was not definitively described until around 1820 [28 p. 22]. Whytt thought that diseases of the nerve system were by "*a too great delicacy and sensibility of the whole nervous system*" as well as error functions of certain organs of the body. As evidence of his theory, Whytt mentions blushing of shame, increased saliva secretion by the sight of food, tears, sorrow, etc. A local irritation of the spinal cord (spinal irritation) was the cause of the patient's symptoms via the reflex arcs. Evidence quoted included spinal TB. When a diagnosis had to be established, the doctor would look for signs of irritation, i.e. *tender points* in muscles, soreness between his shoulder blades, etc. The concept was later used by Charcot, who described the so-called hysterogenic zones; and today similar *tender points* are being used in the diagnosis of fibromyalgia. Once the place of the irritation had been found, treatment was begun by local application of various things on the skin or by corrosion burns, suggilation, etc.

In the 1930s, M Hall proposed the idea that the reflex arcs were part of a separate, autonomous spinal nervous system that controlled the activity of all the body's organs [28 p. 70]. Vomiting during pregnancy, for example, could be due to the irritation of a uterine nerve, which via the reflex arc caused vomiting. The German physiologist and pathologist J. Müller argued that the reflexes also went into the brain, and in 1838 A.W. Volkmann formulated the hypothesis that the brain like the spinal cord reflects the received stimuli [28 p. 70]. Irritation of the uterus and internal organs caused hysteria and other mental disorders through a brain reflex. The hypothesis was supported by clinical studies showing that menstrual disorders and other gynaecologic pathology were exceedingly frequent among mentally ill in asylums.

In his textbook from 1857 [28 p. 43], Romberg, who was one of the most important neurologists in the last century, wrote that hysteria was a *reflex neurosis*, which was caused by irritation of the genitals. Women's genitals were more frequently irritated than men's and therefore they had more frequent attacks. Attacks were spreading largely through the sympathetic ganglia than through the spinal canal. Lozenges described the following treatment principles: 1) elimination of reflex irritation by topical treatment of the genitalia, 2) a general reduction of the excitability of the reflex arcs by bathing or similar, 3) a strengthening the patient's will to resist bodily impulses, i.e. spas, abstinence from masturbation, pelvic surgery, including clitoridectomy. Clitoridectomy, which is the removal of the clitoris, is an operation that has been known since antiquity, and in the 18th-19th century, it was used for the treatment of nymphomania, which usually was held to be equivalent to "chronic masturbation". Later in the 19th century, experiments with cauterisation of the clitoris were performed. In Europe this method was discontinued around the turn of the century, but reports of its use in the U.S. have continued up to the First World War II.

If one organ could affect another organ somewhere else in the body, the reflex arc also had to go the other way. The disease could therefore also be treated by local treatment elsewhere on the body [28 p. 40]. So simple was the rationale behind treatment.

The French physiologist F. Broussais (1821) believed that the stomach was the seat of emotion. In the last part of the 19th century, some psychiatrists used *intestinal melancholy* as a diagnostic entity, and in many asylums it was common for patients to have an enema upon their admission.

The uterus, the ovaries and the clitoris were the most popular organs in which mental disorders in general and hysteria in particular were believed to be seated. Romberg thought that a hysterical attack could be triggered by pressure on the ovaries. Charcot used ovarian compression in a treatment where constant pressure of the ovaries was applied (Figure. 17.2). A more drastic approach was surgical intervention to remove the source of the disease. Gynaecological surgery aimed at removing the source of the "irritations" and hence at treating the reflex hysteria and real mental diseases began in the 1840s. The first ovariectomy on psychological indication was conducted in 1872 by A. Hegaret in Freiburg and R. Battey, in the USA, respectively. The operation, i.e. removal of normal ovaries in younger women on psychological indication, was called Battey's surgery. It quickly spread in the Anglo-Saxon world and in Central Europe during the 1870s and 1880's. In the late 1890s, it was rare in Europe, whereas in the U.S., it continued well into the 20th century.

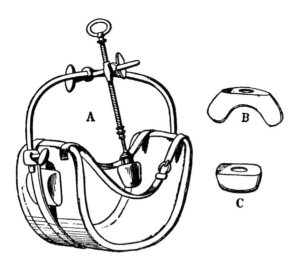

Figure 17.2. Ovary compressor [252]

The reflex theory was not only widespread among gynaecologists, but also found fertile ground among psychiatrists, and the period 1850-1900 saw an entire school of psychiatrists and gynaecologists who believed that women's internal bodies could make them mad and that the best cure therefore was gynaecological surgery [27 p. 69]. Some asylums, especially in the U.S., even had rooms for surgery, and gynaecologists were hired to perform the interventions. In 1884 A. Hegaret declared that the gynaecologist is the "link between somatics and neuropathology".

Towards the end of the 19th century, a widespread theory held that the female pelvic organs could cause mental disorders, i.e. psychoses were considered to be a genital reflex. However, it is questionable whether this theory gained a foothold in Denmark, and no references to these beliefs may be found in elderly Danish text books [256;.257].

A widespread hypothesis derived from the reflex theory in the late 19th century was that irritation of the nasal mucosa was able to cause neurosis. W. Hack from Freiburg claimed that the nasal mucosa was both the end and the start point of reflex arcs, representing the entire body including the brain and uterus. As "evidence" he claimed that diseases of various organs could cause oedema of the nasal mucosa, and as "proof" of this connection he argued that the nasal mucosa became swollen during arousal. It was also argued that a bad cold could lead to cerebral neurasthenia.

In the late 19th century, many neurologists, gynaecologists and ear-nose-throat doctors were preoccupied with finding the anatomical basis for these nasal reflexes, e.g. through the trigeminal nerve. W. Fleiss, who was a practicing doctor in Berlin and a good friend of Freud, was one of the foremost proponents of the nasal reflex theory. He identified genital and abdominal mucosal areas and used stimulation with cocaine, *cauterising* and even surgery to treat for example – "uterohysterical" symptoms and menstrual disorders. Freud had himself been treated in this way and used the diagnosis with his own patients. Nasal treatment according to Fleiss' theory was being used in Germany up to World War II.

Reflex theory and particularly the more dubious theory like the nasal reflex hypothesis may seem ludicrous in our days, but their similarity with for example zonal therapy, which has many supporters, however, is striking.

Hysteria as a psychological/neurological disorder

Although Hippocrates localised mental disorders in the brain, he believed that hysteria was a disorder of uterine origin. Both he and Galen regarded hysteria as a tangible, concrete and logical response to a transient organic imbalance in the body which was primarily due to enforced sexual abstinence. The sexual act was regarded as a purely physical phenomenon, and therefore the effects of abstinence were purely physical by nature [252 p. 42].

In the 15th and the 16th century, there were many followers of Plato's idea that the soul was divided into three parts and that each part had a seat in a separate organ. The brain was the "animal faculty", the heart the "vital faculty" and the liver "nature's faculty". The British doctor E. Jordan in 1603 believed that the primary seat of hysteria was in the "animal faculty", i.e. the head, although the other "faculties" and "sympathy" between them also had some responsibility, though to a lesser degree. He also believed that disturbances of the soul caused hysteria [252 p. 122]. In 1618, the Frenchman C. Piso located the cause of hysteria to the brain. In 1648, Willis, one of the fathers of neurology, believed that hysterical bouts as well as other attacks were due to an "animal spirit localised in the brain, which was ready to explode" [252 p. 132]. The idea that the cause of hysteria is localised in the brain was thus proposed very early in history. However, the soul or the mental processes were not necessarily located to the brain. As outlined above, in reflex theory, the brain was just one among several organs that could affect each other through nerve connections in the spinal canal. The system worked quite mechanically, independently of the will.

Organic brain disorder

In 1836 J. Friederich wrote: *"Psychic diseases do not originate in the first instance in the mind but in a material abnormality, which results in abnormal expression of the individual psychic functions"*, i.e. mental illness is nothing more than a symptom of cerebral disorder, which he believed could be hereditary.

The German professor Wilhelm Griesinger (1817-68) [28 pp. 209-10] became the spokesman of "organic" psychiatry, which was completely dominant in German psychiatry and peaked during 1860-1900. The prevailing trend in psychiatry was that mental disorders were due to anatomical changes and physiological disturbances in the brain. The general belief was that there were no actual differences between neurological and psychiatric disorders, and that that they were merely different manifestations of organic changes in the brain. In other words, mental suffering was part of the neurological disease spectrum. Many of the prominent psychiatrists were therefore interested in neuroanatomy and sought to correlate psychopathological observations with anatomical changes.

However, W. Griesinger had not included hysteria as a genuine mental suffering since he based the diagnosis on a) a hereditary disposition, b) previous bouts of globus hysteria, cramps, sensory disturbances, paralysis and c) a local genitalia disorder. He insisted that all diseases of the uterus, ovaries and vagina were inclined to be followed by hysteria, which, in turn, could gradually evolve into mental illness [252 p. 194].

In France, the neurologist Charcot, who worked at the Salpêtrière Hospital in Paris, held a dominant role in the latter half of the 19th century. Charcot described several neurological disorders and believed, like other contemporaries, that hysteria was a neurological disorder of organic origin, inherited and not a psychiatric disorder [28 p. 7; 253 p. 23; 254 p. 67]. To treat hysteria, he therefore applied methods which had proved effective in other neurological disorders, i.e. careful clinical examination with registration of clinical and paraclinical findings and correlation of these findings to structural changes. He managed, however, never to demonstrate such organic change in hysteria. Charcot believed that the symptom picture in hysteria was rather uniform from patient to patient, and he described three types of symptoms characteristic of hysteria, namely 1) sensory disturbances, e.g. hemianaesthesia and other sensitivity disturbances, 2) disturbance of the senses, e.g. restricted field of vision, deafness and 3) motor disturbances, e.g. aphonia, paralysis and generalised bouts with *arc de cercle* [252]. These pseudo-neurological symptoms have since occupied a special position in the history of hysteria and Guze called them "classical" conversion symptoms [258;259]. He described tenderness of the ovaries as a distinctive feature, but there could be other "hysterogenic" zones in the body, i.e. areas which when touched could cause an attack to begin or to stop, respectively (Figure 17.3). Much of the attention paid to Charcot's theory of hysteria was rooted in his clinical demonstrations and lectures, which resembled theatre more than teaching [28].

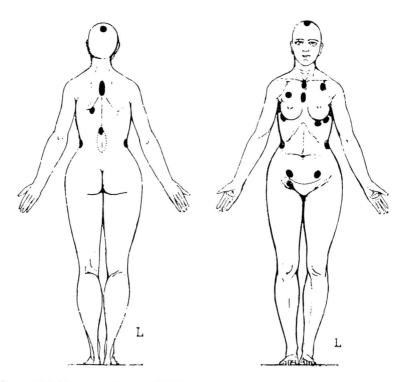

Figure 17.3 Hysterogenic zones [252]

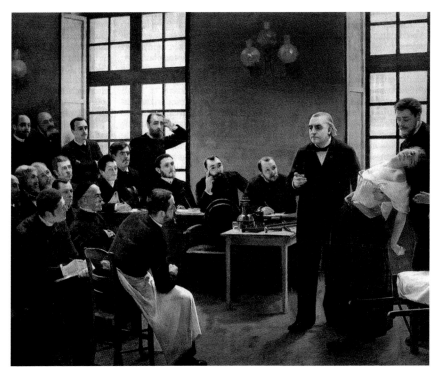

Figure 17.4 Charcot demonstrates the treatment of hysteria in 1886 [252]

Mental illness

Charcot (Figure 17.4) and especially two of his students, Janet and Freud, are generally seen as those who first described hysteria as a mental disorder. This is, however, far from correct. T. Syndenham included hysteria as a disease of the mind and focused on the psychological symptoms accompanying the physical symptoms. However, he had not quite abandoned the idea of the animal spirit as the cause of hysteria [252 p. 142]. Pinel, who is considered one of the modern founders of psychiatry (about 1800), believed that the reason for hysteria was moral or mental. He described a hereditary predisposition to emotional instability. Tantalising speech and reading, abuse of sexual pleasure or, opposite, prolonged abstinence after a rich sex life, were triggering factors.

The English doctor Carter (1828-1918) described hysteria on the basis of a psychodynamic thinking long before Freud was born. According to Veith [252 p. 199], there is so much overlapping between Carter's and Freud's descriptions of psychodynamics that it seems an unlikely coincidence. Carter even described the principles and rationale of psychotherapy, which he termed "moral therapy". In Germany Möbius and Strümpell had similar thoughts about the use of "moral therapy". The idea that hysteria was a mental rather than a neurological disorder achieved its breakthrough in the 1890s. It is difficult to identify a single person who may be credited for this. E. Shorter mentions the Leipzig school with P.J. Möbius, A. Strümpell and E. Kraepelin as the most important persons [28 pp. 239-244]. In particular, Kraeplin's classification of mental disorders was highly important in the classification of hysteria as a mental disorder.

Psychoanalysis

Psychoanalysis arose on the basis of Freud's interest in hysteria. Fenichel [260 p. 230] writes that *"…the psychoanalytic method was discovered, tested, and perfected through the study of hysterical patients; the technique of psycho-analysis still remains most easily applicable to cases of hysteria and it is psycho-analytic treatment of hysteria that continues to yield the best therapeutic results"*.

In Freud and Breuer's "Studies in Hysteria" from 1895, both *physically acquired hysteria* and *dispositional hysteria* are mentioned. The mechanism behind *traumatic hysteria* is that a mental trauma to which a person does not react in a given situation can later be reflected in physical symptoms as a defence against the knowledge of that which was suppressed, e.g. *"… a painful emotion arising during a meal but suppressed at the time, and then producing nausea and vomiting which persists for months in the form of hys-terical vomiting"* [261 p. 4]. The conversion process in this form is almost described as a conditional reflex.

The hypothesis about the conversion process, i.e. the mechanism whereby physical symptoms are generated by hysteria, has by and large remained unchanged until the present day. Freud defined the neuroses not based on the symptom register but on causality. The hysterical neurosis was rooted in the assumption that it was due to a conversion mechanism, i.e. the physical symptoms were a defence mechanism against the knowledge of an inner conflict, and the symptom was a direct symbolic presentation of that internal conflict [260 p. 217].

The hypotheses about the contents of the underlying conflicts and psychodynamic mechanisms were strengthened and modified by Freud in the following years and led to the development of psychoanalytic theory. Through his analysis of hysterical patients he thus found that the repressed traumatic childhood experiences were often of a sexual nature. Specifically, he found that patients frequently presented fantasies of sexual abuse in childhood committed by close persons. This meant that Freud developed the hypothesis of the Oedipus complex, which was a core element of the psychoanalytic theory of the causes of neuroses.

Freudian ideas about conversion hysteria had an exceedingly great impact, and the causal nature of the conversion mechanism has remained virtually unchallenged up to today. This in spite of the fact that the hypothesis actually built on only a few case stories presented by Freud and other contemporaries and no empirical data, wherefore it is difficult to find any scientific support for the classical psychoanalytic theory of the conversion process.

The question is whether the hypothesis builds on an erroneous interpretation of the primary process thinking of poorly structured patients, and whether symptoms are induced by the therapist because of the patient's suggestive potential [260; 260; 263] Freud himself dealt very little with hysteria after his first book.

Since the 1970s, psychoanalytic theories have begun to see major changes. Among emerging theories, Kohut's self-psychology seems especially promising as a psychodynamic frame of reference for the understanding of the somatisation phenomenon, at least in its most severe forms [264;265]. Kohut's basic hypothesis is that anxiety in connection with the threat of defragmentation or disintegration of the self is the deepest form of anxiety a person may experience and that he will therefore do anything in his power to prevent this. According to this model, the physical symptoms can be seen as an unspecific reaction pattern without symbolic significance. This is in better accordance with the available empirically based studies [266].

Hysteria in the 20th century

Many authors and textbooks state that hysteria almost disappeared around the turn of the century after Charcot's death [28; 252; 254]. Many of his pupils like Freud, Janet and Babinski, abandoned the ideas about hysteria shortly after his death and turned to other, more easily definable disorders, and the number of publications about hysteria fell rapidly to almost zero. In the clinic, many psychiatrists even today claim that that hysterical paralysis was only something that existed around the turn of the century. However, the question is whether this is, indeed, true?

Micale [254 pp. 102-106] lists some of the causes of the "disappearance" of hysteria. First, he mentions that an organic basis was found for many of the disorders previously called hysterical. Specifically, he mentions epilepsy. It is undoubtedly true that hysteria had been a too comprehensive diagnosis, and it should be remembered in this connection that Charcot saw hysteria as an organic neurological disorder until a few years before his death. It is a dogma that epilepsy was previously included in hysteria. For example, Hippocrates diagnostically differentiated hysteria from epileptic convulsions by placing a finger on the patient's abdomen. The attack was hysterical if the patient registered pressure and was otherwise epileptic [252 p. 13]. The perception that behind hysteria (and now somatising conditions) lies an undiscovered organic disorder and that the diagnosis to quote Slater [267] is *"a disguise for ignorance and a fertile source of clinical error ..."* now and then surfaces even today and is probably also latent among present-day medical professionals. Doctors apparently find it difficult to fit the seemingly unexplainable causal connections in somatisation disorders and mental disorders alike into the approach to patient's characteristic of rigorous medical science.

Another issue mentioned by Micale [254] is the dramatic developments in psychiatric nosology and the classification system with Kraepelin and Bleuler around and after the turn of the century. Many of the disorders that were previously called hysteria were now classified as *precocious dementia* and later as schizophrenia or other kinds of psychoses. A third reason mentioned by Michale is the introduction of psychoneuroses and the emergence of psychoanalysis, which caused hysteria to give way to anxiety neurosis and other neuroses.

Having offered a historical review, E. Shorter [28] proposes another theory about the "disappearance" of hysteria. He does not believe that hysteria as such disappeared, but its symptom picture changed, and patients are now simply hiding behind other diagnoses and indications. He lists two mechanisms to explain this. Firstly, he argues that man has a common *symptom pool* consisting of all existing symptoms. This *symptom pool* is relatively constant, but new symptoms may be added. The second mechanism is that the somatising patient denies any mental genesis to his physical symptoms/disorders. Just around the turn of the century, hysteria was reclassified from being an organic neurological disorder to being a mental disorder (Janet, Freud, Kraepelin). Psychiatric diagnoses have apparently always been seen as stigmatising by both patients and doctors. The patients have therefore sought, predominantly at the unconscious level and helped by physicians, to find other, more acceptable symptom complexes and diagnoses/designations that do not suggest that the disorder has a mental component. In their choice of symptoms, patients and physicians seem to be influenced by what is up in time. Today, for example, *fibromyalgia, chronic fatigue syndrome* and *MCS*, i.e. sensitivity to odours, are popular diagnoses. E. Short speaks about the diagnosis of the month, precisely like the offer of the week in supermarkets. An example of the changes in symptomatology, is that shell shock was very frequent during World War I where it was believed to be organic injury, while these cases were very rare during World War II where shell shock was considered a mental disorder [253].

Doctors, too, are influenced by fashion, and there is a certain degree of exclusivity and prestige associated with being able to show that you keep abreast of developments and master the latest diagnoses. When new syndromes or diagnoses are introduced, they therefore tend to become too expansive and far too inclusive. This dramatically reduces the validity of the diagnosis and it will at some point raise resistance and lead to a counter movement until the diagnosis settles at an appropriate level. This mechanism was very clear in the hysteria diagnosis. Charcot made the diagnosis exceedingly popular in the latter part of the 19th century, and many types of problems were subsumed under this diagnosis. This resulted in a significant opposition to the diagnosis, so after Charcot's death, virtually no doctor with respect for himself would use the diagnosis. This rebound-effect was so strong that the hysteria diagnosis virtually disappeared for some time.

The main reason for the apparent disappearance of hysteria may lie in administrative/organisational matters. In the middle of the 1800s, psychiatry was organised at large psychiatric asylums geographically isolated both from the rest of society and from the rest of medicine. The somatic patients claimed physical disease and were therefore only to limited extent hospitalised at asylum. The disappearance of hysteria can thus be seen as an artefact caused by the fact that psychiatrists do not come into contact with these patients, and the erroneous conclusion is reached that this disorder has disappeared. Even today, psychiatrists are also largely being educated at asylums and receive only little training in diagnosing and treating these disorders. In psychiatric investigations, these patients are therefore often rejected on the grounds that they are not "psychiatric cases", or that no formal psychiatric disorder has been found.

The lack of interest in functional disorders on the part of asylum psychiatry meant that the psychoanalytic theories received no qualified opposition from Freud's time until the 1960s. General psychiatry has seen violent tensions between the different theoretical orientations, e.g. manic-depressive disorder and schizophrenia; tensions that have led to new developments and advances in treatment.

Because psychoanalysis has enjoyed no similar response regarding somatising conditions, progress in this area largely stagnated in the first half of the 20th century.

Psychosomatics

Psychosomatics dealt with the importance of psychological and social factors for physical suffering. Confusion about the concept of psychosomatics has been substantial. The main reason is that in the psychosomatic tradition, no distinction was made between genuine physical disease and functional disorders. Many are thus using the term psychosomatic disorders as a close synonym for functional disorders [28], that is, disorders where the patient presents with medically unexplained physical symptoms.

Historically, two basic theories have shaped the development of psychosomatic theory, namely psychogenesis and holism. The roots of both concepts go back to antiquity. It should be noted that holism, as described here, has nothing to do with the direction alternative medicine denoted "holistic medicine".

Psychogenesis

Baglivi [268] formulated the problem of psychosomatics already in the early 17th century: "Do passions influence on the body, how can they be treated, and, finally, how can the suffering that originate in emotions be cured?" With the advent of psychoanalysis, the theory of psychogenesis took on a new disguise. Freud's own attitude to the hypothesis that the psyche can cause genuine physical disease is not clear, since he only sparingly dealt with the influence of psychological factors on the physical functions and diseases. Psychoanalytic theories and methods achieved much influence on psychosomatic theory through Freud's pupils. Groddeck, Deutsch, Ferenczi and Jeliffe, among others, applied Freudian hypotheses about conversion hysteria to physical suffering. In its most extreme form, it was postulated that any physical suffering was a symbolic representation of an inner mental conflict aimed at solving, rejecting or keeping out of consciousness an already unconscious conflict [269]. As late as in 1967 Angel and Schmale [270] offered the following example of the mechanism: *"Raynaud's disease appears first in the index finger of a woman about to dial the phone and"* tell off *"her mother, and rheumatoid arthritis first in the ankle of a man with the impulse to kick down the door of a rejecting girlfriend".*

Alexander, who was the dominant profile in psychosomatics from the 1930s to the early 1960s, did not share the perception that physical diseases could be explained by the conversion hysteria mechanism [253;271]. He distinguished between organ neuroses, which he called "vegetative neuroses" and conversion hysteria symptoms, but this distinction is vague and speculative, and he did not distinguish between physical symptoms of genuine physical disease and somatising disorders, i.e. disorders where there is no demonstrated organic basis for the symptoms.

Moreover, Alexander [271] assumed that the nature of the emotional conflict, including personality, would determine which organ was attacked. People who were anti-aggressive would have cardiovascular disorders, for instance, because the pent-up anger would stimulate the sympathetic nervous system, while the dependent patient would get asthma, for instance, through a stimulation of the parasympathetic nervous system. This theory is called the specific theory.

Alexander described some chronic physical diseases whose cause remained unknown and for which no effective treatment existed as particularly interesting from a research perspective. These so-called psychosomatic disorders were called "the great seven", or the Chicago Seven, and consisted of *bronchial asthma, rheumatoid arthritis, ulcerative colitis, essential hypertension, hyperthyroidisms, peptic ulcer disease* and *neurodermatitis*. Despite intensive research efforts, a definitive causal relationship between psychological factors and these diseases has not been demonstrated. In addition, the psychoanalytically oriented treatment of organ neuroses fell short in the 1940s and 1950s.

The theory of psychogenesis is still being defended, albeit in a somewhat modified form. The specific theory has been abandoned, even if a non-specific-theory still exists which assumes *"that psychic factors play a nonspecific role in the multifactorial constellation of disorders that cause illness"* [272].

Holism or the biopsychosocial model

This model lived in the shadow of the reductionist psychogenesis theory throughout the 20th century, but it was only in the early 1950s when Wolff [273] formulated the holistic stress model that the main stream in this research field turned away from the theory of psychogenesis. Wolff rejected the psychogenesis theory, pointing out that emotions are part of a person's psycho-physiological reaction to an event or situation rather than the cause of this reaction. The stress model implies that some people are more vulnerable than others to maladaptive physiological reactions and diseases because their learned ability to withstand stress from a variety of psychosocial stimuli is inadequate.

Wolff introduced the epidemiological methodology in psychosomatics and his work inspired an abundance of empirical research. From the 1960s up to today, the importance of a wide range of factors for health and morbidity have been described. Based on our current knowledge, we must conclude that in every disease there is both a physical and a psychological factor, even if either may be entirely dominant. The term psychosomatic disorder is therefore meaningless and obsolete and has been excluded from the ICD-10 [248].

Today, psychosomatics must be regarded as a broad basic research field that methodologically extends from biochemical studies to sociological population studies [274 p. 37]. The disease model on which psychosomatics is based is the biopsychosocial disease model [43].

Somatoform disorders

A new interest in functional disorders developed in connection with the establishment of *general hospital* psychiatry in the U.S., where psychiatrists suddenly came into contact with these patients. The term somatoform disorder was hence introduced into the DSM-III [249] as a general term for a group of mental disorders predominantly manifesting by physical symptoms. This terminology has later been adopted in the ICD-10 [248]. In *somatoform disorders*, the category of *somatization disorders* was introduced as a specific diagnosis used about a group of chronic somatising patients with multiple physical complaints/symptoms. Other diagnostic subgroups of somatoform disorders include hypochondriasis, *somatoform pain disorder* and conversion-/dissociative disorders. Most also classify the related disorders neurasthenia (chronic fatigue syndrome) and *factitious disorders* under the group of functional disorders.

The DSM-III diagnostic system was a decisive break with the previous classification principles, which were dominated by the psychodynamic theory formation where the diagnoses was divided according to hypotheses and assumptions about underlying causal relationships and mechanisms. With the DSM-III, the ambition was, instead, to introduce an empirically based non-theoretical classification system based largely on symptom descriptions and observational data. The diagnosis of somatisation disorder was the prototype in this classification principle.

Somatisation disorder

The main characteristics of somatising patients is that they complain about medically unexplained symptoms, and the main focus in the diagnostic criteria of somatisation disorder was therefore the number and types of physical symptoms, while the emotional and cognitive complaints were largely neglected.

In order to be able to understand this preoccupation with physical symptoms, it is necessary to look at the medical tradition [255]. The years after the Middle Ages saw a return to Hippocrates' basic scientific principles, where the basic thesis was that any disease had a natural and not a supernatural cause. Efforts were therefore made to determine the cause of disease which was a precondition for rational treatment. All symptoms and clinical findings were carefully registered accordingly and efforts were made to correlate these findings with any anatomical and/or pathophysiological changes. This method, which somewhat condescendingly has been called the "mechanical error model", proved very effective and led to the empirical scientific tradition we see today. The empirical method demonstrated its strength throughout the 19th century when many new diseases were described.

Purtell et al. [275] from St. Louis in the United States resumed the empirical and nosological tradition from the past century when they carefully described 50 patients who had undergone numerous tests without any explanation for their physical complaints being found. Based on this study and a study by Robins and O'Neal [276], Perly and Guze [258;259] in the 1960s constructed the first diagnostic criteria for hysteria, which was later renamed Briquet's syndrome. The patients had to have at least 20 symptoms from a total list of 58 symptoms from nine of ten different organ systems. These criteria included psychiatric symptoms like anxiety, depression and suicide as well as physical symptoms. To avoid overlap with other psychiatric disorder criteria, the criteria were later modified in the sense that all psychiatric symptoms were eliminated which left a total of 37 symptoms [135;277;278]. The criteria for men and women were differentiated, so that men should present 12 complaints and women 14. The syndrome was renamed *somatization disorder* and has been part of the DSM system since the DSM-III was issued. The principles have basically remained unchanged in later editions of the DSM. In the latest DSM-IV, a specific number of symptoms from four symptom groups are required.

Hypochondriasis

The term *hypochondria* was used by Hippocrates about the anatomical region that is located under the curvature. Later, Galen used the term hypochondria to designate a morbid disorder characterised by indigestion problems with flatulence, abdominal pain, nervous anxiety and depression. The condition was believed to be caused by arthritic changes in the pelvic organs, gastrointestinal tract, liver, spleen, etc. The mental symptoms were attributed to an effect of a body fluid on the brain [279]. Early in history, hysteria was often perceived as a uterine variant of hypochondriasis. Thus, Sydenham considered hypochondriasis to be the male counterpart to hysteria in women [280], a view which prevailed until about 1900 [252 pp. 242-243]. In the 18th century, hypochondria was perceived as a fashionable disorder in Britain associated with the English lifestyle.

Hypochondriasis was thus perceived as a disease of the abdominal organs. Many of the cases of hypochondria from the 19th century can today be classified as well-defined physical diseases, which were unknown at the time. Therefore, there is only a partial overlap between the early use of the term and our current understanding of this disorder. The term only achieved its modern sense, i.e. an exaggerated fear of physical disease, with Feuchtersleben in the first part of the 19th century [252 p. 184 and 189] and with Gillespie in the Anglo-Saxon world of Gillespie in 1928.

Hypochondriac worries are frequent in a variety of mental disorders of both psychotic and non-psychotic nature. In the last century, it was thought that hypochondria was the precursor to melancholia (depression) and dementia praecox (schizophrenia). Melancholy was believed in early history to be caused by a disturbance in the black bile, i.e. the cause of the disturbance was localised to the same anatomical region as hypochondria. This may be one of the reasons why the link between depression and hypochondria has attracted interest. Right up to the present day, the existence of hypochondria as a separate diagnostic entity has been called into question, as has the question whether it is always secondary to another mental disorder. Kenyon [249,250] proposed dividing hypochondriasis into a primary or essential form and a secondary type.

Beard's introduction of neurasthenia almost completely engulfed the hypochondria diagnosis. From around the 19th century and until a renewed interest arose in the 1960s, this condition was only sparsely described in the literature because hypochondria was considered a manifestation of neurasthenia [279].

Syndrome diagnoses

Throughout history, a number of different syndrome descriptions have been introduced, but it is beyond the scope of this book to review their history. However, two diagnoses attract considerable interest even today, chronic fatigue syndrome and fibromyalgia, so they will be briefly described.

Neurasthenia and chronic fatigue syndrome (CFS)

In 1880, the New York doctor G. Beard [282;283] introduced the diagnosis of neurasthenia which was characterised by a symptom constellation of muscle weakness, fatigue and pain accompanied by various other physical and mental symptoms. Beard believed that the disorder had to have an organic pathogenesis. The diagnosis quickly became popular throughout the Western world, and it was the most frequently used diagnosis within neuropathology and psychopathology by the 19th century [28;283]. The diagnosis was particularly frequent among middle-class women, and since women were often bed-bound, they were popularly referred to as couch cases.

The popularity of the diagnosis abated in the early years of World War I and it was rarely diagnosed between the two wars [282;283]. This period is therefore referred to as the first wave of chronic fatigue syndrome or neurasthenia. Tiredness or fatigue is a common symptom that can be caused by a variety of disorders. Since the diagnostic possibilities for excluding various organic causes of fatigue were rudimentary, and mental disorders like depression were little known in the 19 century. Many of these cases of neurasthenia would today undoubtedly be considered as undiagnosed physical diseases or mental disorders. These cases are not just undiagnosed physical diseases as evidenced by the many case reports describing successful therapy by treatments that today would be seen as a placebo treatment, e.g. magnetism and hypnotism.

The story behind what is presently termed chronic fatigue syndrome, i.e. the second wave, takes its starting point in multiple independent events [283]. In 1934 there was an epidemic of severe fatigue and muscle pain among 198 employees at the Los Angeles County General Hospital. The cause was attributed to "atypical poliomyelitis". This epidemic was the prototype of later epidemics, and during the 1950s and 1960s a series of epidemics with epidemic neuromyasthenia were described, which we suspect today were due to an unknown viral infection.

In 1968, it was demonstrated that the disease infectious mononucleosis was caused by Epstein-Barr virus, and it was hence believed that the cause of neuromyasthenia had been found. It turned out, however, that a large part of the population had a positive reaction to Epstein-Barrs virus, and that the correlation between haematologically verified chronic EBV and chronic fatigue syndrome was weak. In 1988, Holmes et al. [285] therefore introduced the designation *chronic fatigue syndrome* (CFS).

In England, the term *myalgic encephalomyelitis* (ME) is also used to describe the same symptom picture. This term originates in an epidemic at the Royal Free Hospital in London in 1955 where patients complained of muscle pain, depression and fatigue of unknown reason [283]. The symptoms were attributed to a brain infection.

In 1988, the American Centers for Disease Control (CDC) [285;286] established certain criteria for CFS. Since these criteria were seen as very restrictive, less restrictive criteria have later been set up and a separate *post-infectious fatigue syndrome* has been identified [287]. The terms are today being used about patients who complain of chronic physical and mental fatigue/exhaustion accompanied by a number of other symptoms, such as muscle pain, where no organic basis can be demonstrated, and where the patient has a significantly reduced ability to function [288].

Fibromyalgia

The description of cases with muscle pain with no organic basis goes back to the early 19th century. In 1904, the British neurologist W. Bowers introduced the term fibrositis to designate diffuse pain for which an organic basis could not be detected. Until the late 1960s, fibrositis was considered a psychosomatic rheumatologic disorder of mixed psychogenic and somatoform genesis. Around 1970, focus turned towards rheumatism and the patient's subjective pain complaints and "emotional symptoms", but with negative organic findings [283].

Disordo factitius and Münchhausen's syndrome

Disordo factitius (*factitious* = false or inauthentic) means deliberate imitation or even added disease where the person's own role is denied. Reports about disordo factitius go a long way back in time. Wierus [290], who lived in the 17th century, described how a woman complained that she was daily vomiting pieces of cloth that had been stuffed into her stomach by the devil. Carter describes [290] *simulative complication* of hysteria with simulated hematemesis and haemoptysis caused by leeches in the mouth, swelling due to tight bandages, wounds due to scratching, etc. One of history's most famous cases of *disordo factitius* is provided by Rachel Hertz, who was called the Needle Virgin [291]. She lived in the early 1800s and got this nickname because over a number of years, a total of 389 needles were removed from her body which it was believed she had ingested due to delirium. Rachel Hertz was treated by Herholdt who became internationally renowned for his descriptions of the patient's mysterious disorder. After some years, it was revealed that the symptoms were self-induced, and that the many unnatural findings were caused by her manipulation with paraclinical tests, among others.

Until around the turn of the century, it was not usual to distinguish between a conscious and an unconscious level, and this may be one of the reasons why we historically have done very little to distinguish between *disordo factitius* and hysteria. On the other hand, more attention has been paid to a distinction between these disorders and simulation [252; 256; 292 p. 21; 226 pp. 504-505]. Disordo factitius has apparently been considered a form of hysteria where the deliberate acts are explained as having been committed in a kind of drowsy condition [293]. This attitude has meant that many patients with *disordo factitius* have been regarded as simple simulants, since it was quite obvious that they had not been in a drowsy condition. They have consequently often been treated as simulants or cheaters, which in extreme cases has resulted in prosecution and prison [294].

Any search in modern Danish psychiatric textbooks for *disordo factitius* is in vain. However, the term pathomime which can be considered a subtype of *disordo factitius* is found, designating that a patient presents with dermatological symptoms. In both the DSM-III-R [295] and the ICD-10 [248], factitious disorder is a separate diagnostic entity.

Discrimination between this disorder and Münchhausen's syndrome is unclear, and the syndrome has been described nearly as a more chronic form of *factitious disorder* [78]. The term Münchhausen's syndrome was introduced by Asher [296]. The German Baron von Münchhausen, who lived in the latter half of the 18th century, was unduly credited for this syndrome. The stories about the Baron, with his fantastic lies, were written by Raspe and are entirely fictional [297]. Raspe never personally knew Baron von Münchhausen, and only the name connects the real Baron with the Baron in the stories. *Simulation* is usually not perceived as an expression of abnormal psychopathology because the phenomenon is widespread. This is exemplified among children who do not want to go to school, or among young people who want to avoid military service. In these cases, there is an obvious motive for the behaviour, which separates simulation from *disordo factitius*. Persons who simulate will make a cost-benefit analysis, i.e. they will weigh the advantage of simulating against the cost of the sick role. Patients with *disordo factitius* do not make such analyses, and their self-inflicted diseases may even be life-threatening, just as there is no limit to what procedures, interventions and physical treatment investigations they are willing to subject themselves to.

References

Reference List

[1]   Kaaya S, Goldberg D, Gask L. Management of somatic presentations of psychiatric illness in general medical settings: evaluation of a new training course for general practitioners. Med Educ 1992;26:138-44.

[2]   Morriss R, Gask L, Ronalds C, Downes-Grainger E, Thompson H, Leese B, et al. Cost-effectiveness of a new treatment for somatized mental disorder taught to GPs. Fam Pract 1998 Apr;15(2):119-25.

[3]   Bowman FM, Goldberg DP, Millar T, Gask L, McGrath G. Improving the skills of established general practitioners: the long- term benefits of group teaching. Med Educ 1992 Jan;26(1):63-8.

[4]   Gask L, Goldberg D, Boardman J, Craig T, Goddard C, Jones O, et al. Training general practitioners to teach psychiatric interviewing skills: an evaluation of group training. Med Educ 1991 Sep;25(5):444-51.

[5]   Gask L, Goldberg D, Porter R, Creed F. The treatment of somatization: evaluation of a teaching package with general practice trainees. J Psychosom Res 1989;33(6):697-703.

[6]   Goldberg D, Gask L, O'Dowd T. The treatment of somatization: teaching techniques of reattribution. J Psychosom Res 1989;33(6):689-95.

[7]   Gask L, Goldberg D, Lesser AL, Millar T. Improving the psychiatric skills of the general practice trainee: an evaluation of a group training course. Med Educ 1988 Mar;22(2):132-8.

[8]   Gask L, McGrath G, Goldberg D, Millar T. Improving the psychiatric skills of established general practitioners: evaluation of group teaching. Med Educ 1987 Jul;21(4):362-8.

[9]   Gask L. Management in primary care. In: Mayou R, Bass C, Sharpe M, editors. Treatment of functional somatic symptoms. Oxford, New York, Tokyo: Oxford University Press; 1995: 391-409.

[10]   Gask L, Usherwood T, Thompson H, Williams B. Evaluation of a training package in the assessment and management of depression in primary care. Med Educ 1998 Mar;32(2):190-8.

[11]   Gask L. Small group interactive techniques utilizing videofeedback. Int J Psychiatry Med 1998;28(1):97-113.

[12]   Wonca. International Classification of Primary Care. ICPC-2-R. 2nd ed. New York: Oxford University Press; 2005.

[13]   Nimnuan C, Rabe-Hesketh S, Wessely S, Hotopf M. How many functional somatic syndromes? J Psychosom Res 2001 Oct;51(4):549-57.

[14]   Wessely S, Nimnuan C, Sharpe M. Functional somatic syndromes: one or many? Lancet 1999 Sep 11;354(9182):936-9.

[15]   Barsky AJ, Borus JF. Functional somatic syndromes. Ann Intern Med 1999 Jun 1;130(11):910-21.

[16]   Aaron LA, Buchwald D. A review of the evidence for overlap among unexplained clinical conditions. Ann Intern Med 2001 May 1;134(9 Pt 2):868-81.

[17]   Fink P. Kronisk somatisering Afdeling for Psykiatrisk Demografi, Psykiatrisk Universitetshospital i Aarhus, Universitet; 1997.

[18]   Bornschein S, Forstl H, Zilker T. Idiopathic environmental intolerances (formerly multiple chemical sensitivity) psychiatric perspectives. J Intern Med 2001 Oct;250(4):309-21.

[19]   Fink P, Toft T, Hansen MS, Ørnbøl E, Olesen F. Symptoms and syndromes of bodily distress: an exploratory study of 978 internal medical, neurological, and primary care patients. Psychosom Med 2007 Jan;69(1):30-9.

[20]   Das-Munshi J, Rubin GJ, Wessely S. Multiple chemical sensitivities: A systematic review of provocation studies. J Allergy Clin Immunol 2006 Dec;118(6):1257-64.

[21]   Fink P, Schröder A. One single diagnosis, Bodily distress syndrome, succeeded to capture ten diagnostic categories of functional somatic syndromes and somatoform disorders. Journal of Psychosomatic Research 2010;68:415-26.

[22]   Fink P, Rosendal M, Lyngså Dam KM, Schröder A. Ny fælles diagnose for funktionelle sygdomme. Ugeskr laeger 2010;172(24):1835-38.

[23]   Schröder A, Fink P. Functional Somatic Syndromes and Somatoform Disorders in Special Psychosomatic Units – Organizational Aspects and Evidence-based Treatment. Psychiatr Clin North Am 34 (2011) 673-687. In press 2011.

[24]   O'Malley PG, Jackson JL, Santoro J, Tomkins G, Balden E, Kroenke K. Antidepressant therapy for unexplained symptoms and symptom syndromes. J Fam Pract 1999 Dec;48(12):980-90.

[25]   Kroenke K, Swindle R. Cognitive-Behavioural Therapy for Somatization and Symptom Syndromes: A Critical Review of Controlled Clinical Trials. Psychother Psychosom 2000 Jul;69(4):205-15.

[26]   Henningsen P, Zipfel S, Herzog W. Management of functional somatic syndromes. Lancet 2007 Mar 17;369(9565):946-55.

[27]   Fink P. From hysteria to somatization: A historical perspective. Nord J Psychiatry 1996;50:353-63.

[28]   Shorter E. From Paralysis to Fatigue. A History of Psychosomatic Illness in the Modern Era. New York, Toronto ect.: The Free Press. Macmillan Inc.; 1992.

[29]   Fink P, Rosendal M. Recent developments in the understanding and management of functional somatic symptoms in primary care. Curr Opin Psychiatry 2008 Mar;21(2):182-8.

[30] Creed F, Guthrie E, Fink P, Henningsen P, Rief W, Sharpe M, et al. Is there a better term than "medically unexplained symptoms"? J Psychosom Res 2010 Jan;68(1):5-8.

[31] Stone J, Wojcik W, Durrance D, Carson A, Lewis S, MacKenzie L, et al. What should we say to patients with symptoms unexplained by disease? The "number needed to offend". BMJ 2002 Dec;21;325(7378):1449-50.

[32] Ekholm O, Kjøller M, Davidsen M, Hesse U, Eriksen L, Christensen AL, et al. Sundhed og sygelighed i Danmark 2005 & udviklingen siden 1987. København: Statens Institut for Folkesundhed; 2006.

[33] Kroenke K, Mangelsdorff AD. Common symptoms in ambulatory care: incidence, evaluation, therapy, and outcome. Am J Med 1989;86:262-6.

[34] Creed F, Barsky A. A systematic review of the epidemiology of somatisation disorder and hypochondriasis. J Psychosom Res 2004 Apr;56(4):391-408.

[35] Wittchen HU, Jacobi F. Size and burden of mental disorders in Europe--a critical review and appraisal of 27 studies. Eur Neuropsychopharmacol 2005 Aug;15(4):357-76.

[36] Fink P, Jensen J, Borgquist L, Brevik JI, Dalgard OS, Sandager I, et al. Psychiatric morbidity in primary public health care. A Nordic multicenter investigation. Part I: Method and prevalence of psychiatric morbidity. Acta Psychiatr Scand 1995;92:409-18.

[37] van der Feltz-Cornelis CM, Lyons JS, Huyse FJ, Campos R, Fink P, Slaets JP. Health services research on mental health in primary care. Int J Psychiatry Med 1997;27(1):1-21.

[38] Toft T, Fink P, Oernboel E, Christensen K, Frostholm L, Olesen F. Mental disorders in primary care: prevalence and co-morbidity among disorders. Results from the functional illness in primary care (FIP) study. Psychol Med 2005 Aug;35(8):1175-84.

[39] Arolt V, Driessen M, Dilling H. The Lübeck General Hospital Study. I: Prevalence of psychiatric disorders in medical and surgical inpatients. Int J Psychiat Clin Pract 1997;1:207-16.

[40] Hansen MS, Fink P, Sondergaard L, Frydenberg M. Mental illness and health care use: a study among new neurological patients. Gen Hosp Psychiatry 2005 Mar;27(2):119-24.

[41] Hansen MS, Fink P, Frydenberg M, Oxhoj M, Sondergaard L, Munk-Jørgensen P. Mental disorders among internal medical inpatients: prevalence, detection, and treatment status. J Psychosom Res 2001 Apr;50(4):199-204.

[42] Fink P, Sorensen L, Engberg M, Holm M, Munk-Jorgensen P. Somatization in primary care. Prevalence, health care utilization, and general practitioner recognition. Psychosomatics 1999 Jul;40(4):330-8.

[43] Goldberg D, Huxley P. Common Mental Disorders. A Bio-Social Model. London: Routledge; 1992.

[44] Katon W, Schulberg H. Epidemiology of depression in primary care. Gen Hosp Psychiatry 1992;14:237-47.

[45]   Munk-Jørgensen P, Fink P, Brevik JI, Dalgard OS, Engberg M, Hansson L, et al. Psychiatric morbidity in primary public health care. A multicentre investigation. Part II: Hidden morbidity and choice of treatment. Acta Psychiatr Scand 1997;95:6-12.

[46]   Üstün TB, Sartorius N. Mental illness in General Health Care, An International Study. Chichester, New York, Brisbane, Toronto, Singapore: John Wiley & Sons; 1995.

[47]   Vedsted P, Fink P, Olesen F, Munk-Jørgensen P. Psychological distress as a predictor of frequent attendance in family practice: a cohort study. Psychosomatics 2001 Sep;42(5):416-22.

[48]   Fink P. Somatization Disorder and Related Disorders. In: Gelder MG, López-Ibor JJ, Andreasen NC, editors. New Oxford Textbook of Psychiatry. Oxford: Oxford University Press; 2000: 1080-8.

[49]   Peveler R, Kilkenny L, Kinmonth AL. Medically unexplained physical symptoms in primary care: a comparison of self-report screening questionnaires and clinical opinion. J Psychosom Res 1997 Mar;42(3):245-52.

[50]   Rosendal M, Bro F, Fink P, Christensen KS, Olesen F. General practioners' diagnosis of somatisation: effect of an educational intervention in a cluster randomised controlled trial. Br J Gen Pract 2003 Dec;53(497):917-22.

[51]   Fink P, Ørnbøl E, Toft T, Sparle KC, Frostholm L, Olesen F. A new, empirically established hypochondriasis diagnosis. Am J Psychiatry 2004 Sep;161(9):1680-91.

[52]   Gureje O, Simon GE, Ustun TB, Goldberg DP. Somatization in cross-cultural perspective: a World Health Organization study in primary care. Am J Psychiatry 1997 Jul;154(7):989-95.

[53]   Kirmayer LJ, Robbins JM. Three forms of somatization in primary care: prevalence, co-occurrence, and sociodemographic characteristics. J Nerv Ment Dis 1991 Nov;179(11):647-55.

[54]   Barsky AJ, Wyshak G, Klerman LG. Transient hypochondriasis. Arch Gen Psychiatry 1990 Aug;47(8):746-52.

[55]   De Waal MW, Arnold IA, Eekhof JA, van Hemert AM. Somatoform disorders in general practice: Prevalence, functional impairment and comorbidity with anxiety and depressive disorders. Br J Psychiatry 2004 Jun;184:470-6.

[56]   Fink P, Hansen MS, Oxhoj ML. The prevalence of somatoform disorders among internal medical inpatients. J Psychosom Res 2004 Apr;56(4):413-8.

[57]   Fink P, Hansen MS, Sondergaard L. Somatoform disorders among first-time referrals to a neurology service. Psychosomatics 2005 Nov;46(6):540-8.

[58]   Schröder A. Syndromes of bodily distress. Assessment and treatment. PhD dissertation Faculty of Health Sciences, Aarhus University, Denmark; 2010.

[59]   Prins JB, van der Meer JW, Bleijenberg G. Chronic fatigue syndrome. Lancet 2006 Jan 28;367(9507):346-55.

[60]   Wessely S. The epidemiology of chronic fatigue syndrome. Epidemiol Rev 1995;17(1):139-51.

[61]   Ranjith G. Epidemiology of chronic fatigue syndrome. Occup Med (Lond) 2005 Jan;55(1):13-9.

[62]   McBeth J, Jones K. Epidemiology of chronic musculoskeletal pain. Best Pract Res Clin Rheumatol 2007 Jun;21(3):403-25.

[63]   Goldenberg DL, Burckhardt C, Crofford L. Management of fibromyalgia syndrome. JAMA 2004 Nov:17;292(19):2388-95.

[64]   Drossman DA, Camilleri M, Mayer EA, Whitehead WE. AGA technical review on irritable bowel syndrome. Gastroenterology 2002 Dec:123(6):2108-31.

[65]   Fink P, Ørnbøl E, Christensen KS. The Outcome of Health Anxiety in Primary Care. A Two-Year Follow-up Study on Health Care Costs and Self-Rated Health. PLoS ONE 2010 Mar 24;5(3):e9873.

[66]   Fink P, Jensen J, Poulsen CS. A study of hospital admissions over time, using longitudinal latent structure analysis. Scand J Soc Med 1993;3:211-9.

[67]   Stenager EN, Svendsen MA, Stenager E. Førtidspension til patienter med syndromsygdomme. Ugeskr laeger 2003;5(165):469-74.

[68]   Feinstein AR. The Blame-X syndrome: Problems and lessons in nosology, spectrum, and etiology. Journal of Clinical Epidemiology 2001;54(5):433-9.

[69]   Simon G, Gater R, Kisely S, Piccinelli M. Somatic symptoms of distress: an international primary care study. Psychosomatic Med 1996 Sep;58(5):481-8.

[70]   Kendell RE. Clinical validity. Psychological med 1989;19(1):45-55.

[71]   Rosendal M, Olesen F, Fink P. Diagnostik og klassifikation af Medicinsk Uforklarede Symptomer i almen praksis. Månedsskr Prakt Lægegern 2006;84(4):403-14.

[72]   Fink P, Rosendal M, Olesen F. Classification of somatization and functional somatic symptoms in primary care. Aust N Z J Psychiatry 2005;39(9):772-81.

[73]   Risør MB. Illness explanations among patients with medically unexplained symptoms – different idioms for different contexts. Health 2009;13(5).

[74]   Hall NM. What spings to mind: An investigation into the neural and phenomenological characteristics of involuntary and voluntary conscious memories Faculty of Health Sciences, University of Aarhus; 2006.

[75]   Eisendrath SJ. Factitious illness: A clarification. Psychosomatics 1984;25:110-7.

[76]   Feldman MD, Ford CV. Patient or pretender. Inside the Strange World of Factitious Disorders. New York,Chichester,Brisbane,Toronto,Singapore: John Wiley & Sons, Inc.; 1994.

[77]   Halligang PW, Bass C, Oakley DA. Malingering and Illness Deception. Oxford: Oxford University Press; 2004.

[78]   Fink P, Jensen J. Clinical characteristics of the Munchausen syndrome. A review and 3 new case histories. Psychother Psychosom 1989;52:164-71.

[79]   Spiro RH. Chronic Factitious illness, Munchausen's syndrom. Arch Gen Psychiatry 1968;18:569-79.

[80]   Bursten B. On Munchausen's syndrome. Arch Gen Psychiatry 1965;13:261-8.

[81]   Pankratz. A review of the Munchausen syndrome. Clin Psychol Rev 1981;1:65-78.

[82]   Ford CV. The Somatizing Disorders. Illness as a Way of Life. New York, Amsterdam, Oxford: Elsevier Biomedical.; 1983.

[83]   Reich P, Gottfried LA. Factitious disorders in a teaching hospital. Ann Intern Med 1983;99:240-7.

[84]   Moss-Morris R, Spence M. To "lump" or to "split" the functional somatic syndromes: can infectious and emotional risk factors differentiate between the onset of chronic fatigue syndrome and irritable bowel syndrome? Psychosom Med 2006 May;68(3):463-9.

[85]   Jenkins DC. New horizons for psychosomatic medicine. Psochosomatic med 1985;47:3-25.

[86]   Kato K, Sullivan PF, Evengard B, Pedersen NL. A population-based twin study of functional somatic syndromes. Psychological med 2009 Mar;39(3):497-505.

[87]   Clauw DJ. Potential mechanisms in chemical intolerance and related conditions. Ann N Y Acad Sci 2001 Mar;933:235-53.

[88]   BENTALL RP, POWELL PAUL, NYE FJ, EDWARDS RHT. Predictors of response to treatment for chronic fatigue syndrome. The British Journal of Psychiatry 2002 Sep 1;181(3):248-52.

[89]   McDaniel S, Campbell T, Seaburn D. Somatic Fixation in Patients and Physicians: A Biopsychosocial Approach. Family Systems Medicine 1989;7(1):5-16.

[90]   Martin RL, Cloninger CR, Guze SB. The evaluation of Diagnostic Concordance in Follow-up studies: II. A Blind, prospective Follow-up of Female Criminals. J Psychiatr Res 1979;15:107-25.

[91]   Guze SB, Cloninger CR, Martin RL, Clayton PJ. A Follow-up and Family Study of Briquet's Syndrome. Br J Psych 1986;149:17-23.

[92]   Deary V, Chalder T, Sharpe M. The cognitive behavioural model of medically unexplained symptoms: a theoretical and empirical review. Clin Psychol Rev 2007 Oct;27(7):781-97.

[93]   Rief W, Shaw R, Fichter MM. Elevated levels of psychophysiological arousal and cortisol in patients with somatization syndrome [In Process Citation]. Psychosomatic Med 1998 Mar;60(2):198-203.

[94]   Kuchinad A, Schweinhardt P, Seminowicz DA, Wood PB, Chizh BA, Bushnell MC. Accelerated brain gray matter loss in fibromyalgia patients: premature aging of the brain? J Neurosci 2007 Apr 11;27(15):4004-7.

[95]   De Lange FP, Kalkman JS, Bleijenberg G, Hagoort P, van der Meer JW, Toni I. Gray matter volume reduction in the chronic fatigue syndrome. Neuroimage 2005 Jul 1;26(3):777-81.

[96]   Burgmer M, Gaubitz M, Konrad C, Wrenger M, Hilgart S, Heuft G, et al. Decreased Gray Matter Volumes in the Cingulo-Frontal Cortex and the Amygdala in Patients With Fibromyalgia. Psychosomatic Med 2009 May 4.

[97]   Valet M, Gundel H, Sprenger T, Sorg C, Muhlau M, Zimmer C, et al. Patients with pain disorder show gray-matter loss in pain-processing structures: a voxel-based morphometric study. Psychosomatic Med 2009 Jan;71(1):49-56.

[98]   Kuzminskyte R. Impaired sensory processing in patients with multiple somatic symptoms. PhD dissertation 2008.

[99]   Wood PB. Neuroimaging in functional somatic syndromes. Int Rev Neurobiol 2005;67:119-63.

[100]   Dimsdale JE, Dantzer R. A biological substrate for somatoform disorders: importance of pathophysiology. Psychosomatic Med 2007 Dec;69(9):850-4.

[101]   Maletic V, Raison CL. Neurobiology of depression, fibromyalgia and neuropathic pain. Front Biosci 2009 Jun 1;14:5291-338.:5291-338.

[102]   Johnson S, Summers J, Pridmore S. Changes to somatosensory detection and pain thresholds following high frequency repetitive TMS of the motor cortex in individuals suffering from chronic pain. Pain 2006 Jul;123(1-2):187-92.

[103]   Pujol J, Lopez-Sola M, Ortiz H, Vilanova JC, Harrison BJ, Yucel M, et al. Mapping brain response to pain in fibromyalgia patients using temporal analysis of FMRI. PLoS ONE 2009;4(4):e5224.

[104]   Schweinhardt P, Sauro KM, Bushnell MC. Fibromyalgia: A Disorder of the Brain? Neuroscientist 2008 Feb 12.

[105]   Rief W, Barsky AJ. Psychobiological perspectives on somatoform disorders. Psychoneuroendocrinology 2005 Jun 13;30(10):996-1002.

[106]   Bonifazi M, Lisa SA, Cambiaggi C, Felici A, Grasso G, Lodi L, et al. Changes in salivary cortisol and corticosteroid receptor-alpha mRNA expression following a 3-week multidisciplinary treatment program in patients with fibromyalgia. Psychoneuroendocrinology 2006 Oct;31(9):1076-86.

[107]   McBeth J, Chiu YH, Silman AJ, Ray D, Morriss R, Dickens C, et al. Hypothalamic-pituitary-adrenal stress axis function and the relationship with chronic widespread pain and its antecedents. Arthritis Res Ther 2005;7(5):R992-R1000.

[108]   Chang L, Berman S, Mayer EA, Suyenobu B, Derbyshire S, Naliboff B, et al. Brain responses to visceral and somatic stimuli in patients with irritable bowel syndrome with and without fibromyalgia. Am J Gastroenterol 2003 Jun;98(6):1354-61.

[109]   Chang L. Brain responses to visceral and somatic stimuli in irritable bowel syndrome: a central nervous system disorder? Gastroenterol Clin North Am 2005 Jun;34(2):271-9.

[110]   Song GH, Venkatraman V, Ho KY, Chee MW, Yeoh KG, Wilder-Smith CH. Cortical effects of anticipation and endogenous modulation of visceral pain assessed by functional brain MRI in irritable bowel syndrome patients and healthy controls. Pain 2006 Dec 15;126(1-3):79-90.

[111]   Price DD, Zhou Q, Moshiree B, Robinson ME, Verne GN. Peripheral and central contributions to hyperalgesia in irritable bowel syndrome. J Pain 2006 Aug;7(8):529-35.

[112]   Rossel P, Pedersen P, Niddam D, rendt-Nielsen L, Chen ACN, Drewes AM. Cerebral response to electric stimulation of the colon and abdominal skin in healthy subjects and patients with irritable bowel syndrome. Scandinavian Journal of Gastroenterology 2001;36(12):1259-66.

[113]   Staud R, Spaeth M. Psychophysical and neurochemical abnormalities of pain processing in fibromyalgia. CNS Spectr 2008 Mar;13(3 Suppl 5):12-7.

[114] Wood PB, Schweinhardt P, Jaeger E, Dagher A, Hakyemez H, Rabiner EA, et al. Fibromyalgia patients show an abnormal dopamine response to pain. Eur J Neurosci 2007 Jun;25(12):3576-82.

[115] Wood PB, Glabus MF, Simpson R, Patterson JC. Changes in Gray Matter Density in Fibromyalgia: Correlation With Dopamine Metabolism. J Pain 2009 Apr 22.

[116] Gundel H, Valet M, Sorg C, Huber D, Zimmer C, Sprenger T, et al. Altered cerebral response to noxious heat stimulation in patients with somatoform pain disorder. Pain 2008 Jul 15;137(2):413-21.

[117] Rief W, Pilger F, Ihle D, Verkerk R, Scharpe S, Maes M. Psychobiological aspects of somatoform disorders: contributions of monoaminergic transmitter systems. Neuropsychobiology 2004;49(1):24-9.

[118] Miller L. Neuropsychological concepts of somatoform disorders. Int J Psychiatry Med 1984;14(1):31-46.

[119] James L, Gordon E, Kraiuhin C, Meares R. Selective attention and auditory event-related potentials in somatization disorder. Compr Psychiatry 1989;Jan-Feb;30(1):84-9.

[120] Rief W, Broadbent E. Explaining medically unexplained symptoms-models and mechanisms. Clin Psychol Rev 2007;27(7):821-41.

[121] Yunus MB. Fibromyalgia and overlapping disorders: the unifying concept of central sensitivity syndromes. Semin Arthritis Rheum 2007 Jun;36(6):339-56.

[122] Yunus MB. Central Sensitivity Syndromes: A New Paradigm and Group Nosology for Fibromyalgia and Overlapping Conditions, and the Related Issue of Disease versus Illness. Semin Arthritis Rheum 2008 Jan 11.

[123] Bradley LA. Pathophysiologic mechanisms of fibromyalgia and its related disorders. J Clin Psychiatry 2008;69 Suppl 2:6-13.:6-13.

[124] Botega NJ, Pereira WA, Bio MR, Garcia Junior C, Zomignani MA. Psychiatric morbidity among medical in-patients: a standardized assessment (GHQ-12 and CIS-R) using 'lay' interviewers in a Brazilian hospital. Soc Psychiatry Psychiatr Epidemiol 1995;30(3):127-31.

[125] Woolf CJ, Salter MW. Neuronal plasticity: increasing the gain in pain. Science 2000 Jun 9;288(5472):1765-9.

[126] Mertz H. Role of the brain and sensory pathways in gastrointestinal sensory disorders in humans. Gut 2002 Jul;51 Suppl 1:i29-i33.

[127] Aguggia M. Neurophysiology of pain. Neurol Sci 2003 May;24 Suppl 2:S57-S60.

[128] Browning M, Fletcher P, Sharpe M. Can neuroimaging help us to understand and classify somatoform disorders? A systematic and critical review. Psychosomatic Med 2011 Feb;73(2):173-84.

[129] Jones AK, Kulkarni B, Derbyshire SW. Functional imaging of pain perception. Curr Rheumatol Rep 2002 Aug;4(4):329-33.

[130] Price J, Leaver L. Beginning treatment. In: Mayou R, Sharpe M, Carson A, editors. ABC of Psychological Medicine.London: BMJ Books; 2003: 4-6.

[131] Quill TE. Somatization Disorder. One of Medicine's Blind Spots. JAMA 1985;254:254.

[132] Crimlisk HL, Bhatia K, Cope H, David A, Marsden CD, Ron MA. Slater revisited: 6 year follow up study of patients with medically unexplained motor symptoms. BMJ 1998 Feb 21;316(7131):582-6.

[133] Wilson A, Hickie I, Lloyd A, Hadzi-Pavlovic D, Boughton C, Dwyer J, et al. Longitudinal study of outcome of chronic fatigue syndrome. BMJ 1994 Mar 19;308(6931):756-9.

[134] Stone J, Smyth R, Carson A, Lewis S, Prescott R, Warlow C, et al. Systematic review of misdiagnosis of conversion symptoms and "hysteria". BMJ 2005 Oct 29;331(7523):989.

[135] Bass C. Somatization:Physical Symptoms & Psychological Illness. 1 ed. Oxford: Blackwell Scientific Publications; 1990.

[136] Williamson P, Beitman BD, Katon W. Beliefs that foster physician avoidance of psychosocial aspects of health care. J Fam Pract 1981;13:999-1003.

[137] Bass C, Peveler R, House A. Somatoform disorders: severe psychiatric illnesses neglected by psychiatrists. Br J Psychiatry 2001 Jul;179:11-4.

[138] Creed F. Should general psychiatry ignore somatization and hypochondriasis? World Psychiatry 2006 Oct;5(3):146-50.

[139] Lucock MP, Morley S, White C, Peake MD. Responses of consecutive patients to reassurance after gastroscopy: results of self administered questionnaire survey. BMJ 1997 Sep 6;315(7108):572-5.

[140] Hansen HS. Medically unexplained symptoms in primary care – a mixed method study of diagnosis. PhD dissertation. The Research Clinic for Functional Disorders and Psychosomatics / The Research Unit for General Practice. Faculty of Health Sciences, Aarhus University; 2009.

[141] Balint M. The doctor, his patients and the illness. London: Pitman Medical; 1957.

[142] Marchant-Haycox S, Salmon P. Patients' and doctors' strategies in consultations with unexplained symptoms. Interactions of gynecologists with women presenting menstrual problems. Psychosomatics 1997 Sep;38(5):440-50.

[143] Salmon P. Conflict, collusion or collaboration in consultations about medically unexplained symptoms: The need for a curriculum of medical explanation. Patient Educ Couns 2007 Apr 9.

[144] Salmon P, Wissow L, Carroll J, Ring A, Humphris GM, Davies JC, et al. Doctors' attachment style and their inclination to propose somatic interventions for medically unexplained symptoms. Gen Hosp Psychiatry 2008 Mar;30(2):104-11.

[145] Salmon P, Humphris GM, Ring A, Davies JC, Dowrick CF. Primary care consultations about medically unexplained symptoms: patient presentations and doctor responses that influence the probability of somatic intervention. Psychosomatic Med 2007 Jul;69(6):571-7.

[146] Stern TA, Prager LM, Cremens MC. Autognosis Rounds for Medical House Staff. Psychosomatics 1993;34(1 January-Febuary):1-7.

[147] White J, Levinson W, Roter D. "Oh, by the way …": the closing moments of the medical visit. J Gen Intern Med 1994 Jan;9(1):24-8.

[148] Mechanic D. The Concept of Illness behavior. J Chronic Dis 1961;15:189-94.

[149] Fink P. Psykiatrisk og somatisk comorbiditet. Befolkningens forbrug af hospitals indlæggelser. Institut for psykiatrisk grundforskning. Afdeling for psykiatrisk Demografi. Psykiatrisk hospital i Århus; 1992.

[150] Weinman J, Petrie KJ, Moss-Morris R, Horne R. The Illness Perception Questionnaire: A New Method for Assessing the Cognitive Representation of Illness. Psychology and Health 1996;11:431-45.

[151] Schmidt AJ, Wolfs Takens DJ, Oosterlaan J, van den Hout MA. Psychological mechanisms in hypochondriasis: attention-induced physical symptoms without sensory stimulation. Psychother Psychosom 1994;61:117-20.

[152] Jensen ST, de Fine Olivarius B, Kraft M, Hansen HJ. Familial hemiplegic migraine-areappraisal and a long-term follow-up study. Cephalalgia 1981;1:33-9.

[153] Göthe CJ, Molin CM, Nilsson CG. The Environomental Somatization Syndrome. Psychosomatics 1995;36(1):1-11.

[154] Allen LA, Escobar JI, Lehrer PM, Gara MA, Woolfolk RL. Psychosocial treatments for multiple unexplained physical symptoms: a review of the literature. Psychosom Med 2002 Nov;64(6):939-50.

[155] Toft T. Managing patients with functional somatic symptoms in general practice Faculty of Health Sciences, University of Aarhus, Denmark; 2005.

[156] Kroenke K. Efficacy of treatment for somatoform disorders: a review of randomized controlled trials. Psychosomatic Med 2007 Dec;69(9):881-8.

[157] Whiting P, Bagnall AM, Sowden AJ, Cornell JE, Mulrow CD, Ramirez G. Interventions for the treatment and management of chronic fatigue syndrome: a systematic review. JAMA 2001 Sep 19;286(11):1360-8.

[158] Hauser W, Bernardy K, Uceyler N, Sommer C. Treatment of fibromyalgia syndrome with antidepressants: a meta-analysis. JAMA 2009 Jan 14;301(2):198-209.

[159] Ford AC, Talley NJ, Schoenfeld PS, Quigley EM, Moayyedi P. Efficacy of antidepressants and psychological therapies in irritable bowel syndrome: systematic review and meta-analysis. Gut 2009 Mar;58(3):367-78.

[160] Rahimi R, Nikfar S, Rezaie A, Abdollahi M. Efficacy of tricyclic antidepressants in irritable bowel syndrome: a meta-analysis. World J Gastroenterol 2009 Apr 7;15(13):1548-53.

[161] Jackson JL, O'Malley PG, Kroenke K. Antidepressants and cognitive-behavioral therapy for symptom syndromes. CNS Spectr 2006 Mar;11(3):212-22.

[162] Sumathipala A. What is the evidence for the efficacy of treatments for somatoform disorders? A critical review of previous intervention studies. Psychosomatic Med 2007 Dec;69(9):889-900.

[163] Edmonds M, McGuire H, Price J. Exercise therapy for chronic fatigue syndrome. Cochrane Database Syst Rev 2004;(3):CD003200.

[164] White PD, Goldsmith KA, Johnson AL, Potts L, Walwyn R, DeCesare JC, et al. Comparison of adaptive pacing therapy, cognitive behaviour therapy, graded exercise therapy, and specialist medical care for chronic fatigue syndrome (PACE): a randomised trial. Lancet 2011 Mar 5;377(9768):823-36.

[165] Busch AJ, Barber KA, Overend TJ, Peloso PM, Schachter CL. Exercise for treating fibromyalgia syndrome. Cochrane Database Syst Rev 2007;(4):CD003786.

[166] Hauser W, Klose P, Langhorst J, Moradi B, Steinbach M, Schiltenwolf M, et al. Efficacy of different types of aerobic exercise in fibromyalgia syndrome: a systematic review and meta-analysis of randomised controlled trials. Arthritis Res Ther 2010;12(3):R79.

[167] Donta ST, Clauw DJ, Engel CC, Jr., Williams DA, Barkhuizen A, Taylor T, et al. Cognitive behavioral therapy and aerobic exercise for Gulf War veterans' illnesses: a randomized controlled trial. JAMA 2003 Mar 19;289(11):1396-404.

[168] White PD, Goldsmith KA, Johnson AL, Potts L, Walwyn R, DeCesare JC, et al. Comparison of adaptive pacing therapy, cognitive behaviour therapy, graded exercise therapy, and specialist medical care for chronic fatigue syndrome (PACE): a randomised trial. Lancet 2011 Mar 5;377(9768):823-36.

[169] Price JR, Mitchell E, Tidy E, Hunot V. Cognitive behaviour therapy for chronic fatigue syndrome in adults. Cochrane Database Syst Rev 2008;(3):CD001027.

[170] Glombiewski JA, Sawyer AT, Gutermann J, Koenig K, Rief W, Hofmann SG. Psychological treatments for fibromyalgia: a meta-analysis. Pain 2010 Nov;151(2):280-95.

[171] Bernardy K, Fuber N, Kollner V, Hauser W. Efficacy of cognitive-behavioral therapies in fibromyalgia syndrome – a systematic review and metaanalysis of randomized controlled trials. J Rheumatol 2010 Oct;37(10):1991-2005.

[172] Zijdenbos IL, de Wit NJ, van der Heijden GJ, Rubin G, Quartero AO. Psychological treatments for the management of irritable bowel syndrome. Cochrane Database Syst Rev 2009;(1):CD006442.

[173] Lackner JM, Mesmer C, Morley S, Dowzer C, Hamilton S. Psychological treatments for irritable bowel syndrome: a systematic review and meta-analysis. J Consult Clin Psychol 2004 Dec;72(6):1100-13.

[174] Kisely SR, Campbell LA, Skerritt P, Yelland MJ. Psychological interventions for symptomatic management of non-specific chest pain in patients with normal coronary anatomy. Cochrane Database Syst Rev 2010 Jan;(1):CD004101.

[175] Allen LA, Woolfolk RL, Escobar JI, Gara MA, Hamer RM. Cognitive-behavioral therapy for somatization disorder: a randomized controlled trial. Arch Intern Med 2006 Jul 24;166(14):1512-8.

[176] Kleinstauber M, Witthoft M, Hiller W. Efficacy of short-term psychotherapy for multiple medically unexplained physical symptoms: a meta-analysis. Clin Psychol Rev 2011 Feb;31(1):146-60.

[177] Jackson JL, O'Malley PG, Tomkins G, Balden E, Santoro J, Kroenke K. Treatment of functional gastrointestinal disorders with antidepressant medications: a meta-analysis. Am J Med 2000 Jan;108(1):65-72.

[178] O'Malley PG, Balden E, Tomkins G, Santoro J, Kroenke K, Jackson JL. Treatment of fibromyalgia with antidepressants: a meta-analysis. J Gen Intern Med 2000 Sep;15(9):659-66.

[179] Gormsen L, Jensen TS, Bach FW, Rosenberg R. [Pain and depression]. Ugeskr laeger 2006 May 15;168(20):1967-9.

[180] Hauser W, Schmutzer G, Brahler E, Glaesmer H. A cluster within the continuum of biopsychosocial distress can be labeled "fibromyalgia syndrome"--evidence from a representative German population survey. J Rheumatol 2009 Dec;36(12):2806-12.

[181] Stuart MR. The BATHE Technique in Rakel RE. In: Saunders WB, editor. Saunders Manual of Medical Practice.Philadelphia, PA: 1996: 1108-9.

[182] World Health Organization: Disability Assessment Schedule II. Geneva: World Health Organization; 2005.

[183] Salmon P, Peters S, Stanley I. Patients' perceptions of medical explanations for somatisation disorders: qualitative analysis. BMJ 1999 Feb 6;318(7180):372-6.

[184] Peters S, Stanley I, Rose M, Salmon P. Patients with medically unexplained symptoms: sources of patients' authority and implications for demands on medical care. Soc Sci Med 1998 Feb;46(4-5):559-65.

[185] Dowrick CF, Ring A, Humphris GM, Salmon P. Normalisation of unexplained symptoms by general practitioners: a functional typology. Br J Gen Pract 2004 Mar;54(500):165-70.

[186] Balint M. The Doctor's therapeutic function. Lancet 1965;1177-80.

[187] Schröder A, Rosendal M, Fink P. Kognitiv adfærdsterapi i behandlingen af somatiseringstilstande of funktionelle syndromer. Månedsskr Prakt Lægegern 2007;85:1035-48.

[188] Mynors-Wallis L. Problem-solving treatment: evidence for effectiveness and feasibility in primary care. Int J Psychiatry Med 1996;26(3):249-62.

[189] Wilkinson P, Mynors-Wallis L. Problem-solving therapy in the treatment of unexplained physical symptoms in primary care: a preliminary study. J Psychosom Res 1994 Aug;38(6):591-8.

[190] Rosenberg N. Kognitiv terapi – historie og centrale begreber. Månedsskr Prakt Lægegern 2008;10:10-8.

[191] Graded Exercise Therapy. A self-help guide for those with chronic fatigue syndrome/myalgic encephalomyelitis. St.Bartholomew's Hospital. 2009. Bart's and The London NHS Trust.

[192] Ramchandani PG, Stein A, Hotopf M, Wiles NJ. Early parental and child predictors of recurrent abdominal pain at school age: results of a large population-based study. J Am Acad Child Adolesc Psychiatry 2006 Jun;45(6):729-36.

[193] Walker LS. Pathways between recurrent abdominal pain and adult functional gastrointestinal disorders. J Dev Behav Pediatr 1999 Oct;20(5):320-2.

[194] Garralda ME, Rangel L. Childhood chronic fatigue syndrome. Am J Psychiatry 2001 Jul;158(7):1161.

[195] Lindley KJ, Glaser D, Milla PJ. Consumerism in healthcare can be detrimental to child health: lessons from children with functional abdominal pain. Arch Dis Child 2005 Apr;90(4):335-7.

[196] Crushell E, Rowland M, Doherty M, Gormally S, Harty S, Bourke B, et al. Importance of parental conceptual model of illness in severe recurrent abdominal pain. Pediatrics 2003 Dec;112(6 Pt 1):1368-72.

[197] Garralda ME. Unexplained physical complaints. Child Adolesc Psychiatr Clin N Am 2010 Apr;19(2):199-209, vii.

[198] Rask CU, Olsen EM, Elberling H, Christensen MF, Ornbol E, Fink P, et al. Functional somatic symptoms and associated impairment in 5-7-year-old children: the Copenhagen Child Cohort 2000. Eur J Epidemiol 2009;24(10):625-34.

[199] Garralda ME, Bailey D. Psychosomatic aspects of children's consultations in primary care. Eur Arch Psychiatry Neurol Sci 1987;236(5):319-22.

[200] Huang RC, Palmer LJ, Forbes DA. Prevalence and pattern of childhood abdominal pain in an Australian general practice. J Paediatr Child Health 2000 Aug;36(4):349-53.

[201] Garber J, Walker LS, Zeman J. Somatization symptoms in a community sample of children and adolescents: further validation of The Childrens Somatization Inventory. *Psychological Assessment* 1991; 588-595. Ref Type: Generic

[202] Campo JV, Fritsch SL. Somatization in children and adolescents. J Am Acad Child Adolesc Psychiatry 1994 Nov;33(9):1223-35.

[203] Kotagal P, Costa M, Wyllie E, Wolgamuth B. Paroxysmal nonepileptic events in children and adolescents. Pediatrics 2002 Oct;110(4):e46.

[204] Eminson DM. Medically unexplained symptoms in children and adolescents. Clin Psychol Rev 2007 Jul 17.

[205] Schulte IE, Petermann F. Somatoform disorders: 30 years of debate about criteria! What about children and adolescents? J Psychosom Res 2011 Mar;70(3):218-28.

[206] Rask CU, Elberling H, Skovgaard AM, Thomsen PH, Fink P. Parental-Reported Health Anxiety Symptoms in 5- to 7-Year-Old Children: The Copenhagen Child Cohort CCC 2000. *Psychosomatics* 2011. Ref Type: Generic

[207] Schulte IE, Petermann F. Familial Risk Factors for the Development of Somatoform Symptoms and Disorders in Children and Adolescents: A Systematic Review. Child Psychiatry Hum Dev 2011 May 26.

[208] Janicke DM, Finney JW, Riley AW. Children's health care use: a prospective investigation of factors related to care-seeking. Med Care 2001 Sep;39(9):990-1001.

[209] Schulte IE, Petermann F, Noeker M. Functional abdominal pain in childhood: from etiology to maladaptation. Psychother Psychosom 2010;79(2):73-86.

[210] Campo JV, Fritz G. A management model for pediatric somatization. Psychosomatics 2001 Nov;42(6):467-76.

[211] Garralda ME. Practitioner review: Assessment and management of somatisation in childhood and adolescence: a practical perspective. J Child Psychol Psychiatry 1999 Nov;40(8):1159-67.

[212] Eminson DM. Somatising in children and adolescents. 2. Management and outcomes. *Advances in Psychiatric Treatment* 2001; 388-398. Ref Type: Generic

[213] Walker LS, Garber J. Manual for the Children's Somatization Inventory. 2003. Division of Adolescent Medicine and Behavioral Science, Department of Pediatrics, Vanderbilt University School of Medicine, Nashville. Ref Type: Generic

[214] Husain K, Browne T, Chalder T. A review of psychological models and interventions for medically unexplained somatic symptoms in children. *Child and Adolescent Mental Health* 2008; 2-7. Ref Type: Generic

[215] Crook S, Pakulski J, Waters M. Postmodernization – Change in advance society. London/Newbury Park/New Delhi: Sage Publications; 1992.

[216] Mauss M. Techniques of the body. Economy and Society 1935;(2):70-88.

[217] Blacking J. Towards an anthropology of the body. In: Blacking J, editor. The anthropology of the body. London: 1977.

[218] Winzeler RL. Latah in Southeast Asia. The history and ethnography of a culture-bound syndrome. Cambridge: Cambridge University Press; 1995.

[219] Kleinman AM. Depression, somatization and the "new cross-cultural psychiatry". Social science and medicine 1987;11(24):119-34.

[220] Kleinmann A. Social origins of disease and distress. Depression, neurasthenia and pain in modern China. London: Yale University Press; 1986.

[221] Conrad P. The Medicalization of Society. On the Transformation of Human Conditions into Treatable Disorders. Baltimore: The John Hopkins University Press; 2007.

[222] Honkasalo ML, Lindquist J. An interview with Arthur Kleinman. Ethnos. London: 1997:107-26.

[223] Lieban RW. From illness to symbol and symbol to illness. Social science and medicine 2011;35:183-8.

[224] Kirmayer LJ. Languages of Suffering and Healing: Alexithymia as a Social and Cultural Process. Transcultural Psychiatric Research Review 1987;24:119-1.

[225] Bourdieu P. Site effects. The Weight of The World. Social Suffering in Contemporary Society. Polity Press; 1993.

[226] Helman C. Culture, health and illness. Wright PSG 1984.

[227] Dalsgaard T. "If only I had been in a wheelchair". An anthropological analysis of narratives of sufferers with medically unexplained symptoms. PhD thesis. The Research Clinic for Functional Disorders, Faculty of Health Sciences; 2005.

[228] Risør MB. Healing and recovery as a social process among patients with medically unexplained symptoms (MUS). In: Fainzang S, Hem HE, Risør MB, editors. The Taste for Knowledge: Medical Anthropology Facing Medical Realities. Aarhus Univeristy Press; 2010:131-49.

[229] Ostenfeld-Rosenthal A. Symbolsk healing 'embodied': Krop, mening og spiritualitet i danske helbredelsesritualer. Tidsskrift for Forskning i Sygdom og Samfund 2007;5.

[230] Vohnsen NH. Self-diagnosing with multiple chemical sensitivity – an exploration of the interplay between ecperience and action. Speciale. Afdeling for Antropologi og Etnografi, Aarhus Universitet 2007.

[231] Junge AG. Multiple chemical sensitivity: En antropologisk analyse af, hvordan kropslige erfaringer, kulturelle kategorier og sociale strukturer spiller sammen i oplevelsen af at lide af MCS. Speciale. Afdeling for Antropologi og Etnografi, Aarhus Universitet; 2008.

[232] Mik-Meyer N, Johansen MB. Magtfulde diagnoser og diffuse lidelser. Samfundslitteratur; 2009.

[233] Hellegaard LV. Det er ikke nok at have det dårligt… En empirisk analyse af sygerollens konstruktion i Danmark. Speciale Pædagogisk Antropologi, Danmarks Pædagogiske Universitetsskole; 2008.

[234] Greco M. Illness as a work of thought. London / New York: Routledge; 1998.

[235] Greco M. The question of "humanity": Medical hunmanities and anthroplogical medicine. Einsteinforum, Potsdam 2005.

[236] Greco M. Governmentality and the value of introspection. Invited plenary, Swiss Society for Medical Anthopology, University of Zürich 2004.

[237] Nettleton S, Watt I, O'Malley L, Duffey P. Enigmatic illnesses: Narratives of patients who live with medically unexplained symptoms. Social Theory & Health 2004;2:47-66.

[238] Nettleton S, Watt I, O'Malley L, Duffey P. Understanding the narratives of people who live with medically unexplained illness. Patient Educ Couns 2005 Feb;56(2):205-10.

[239] Peters S, Rogers A, Salmon P, Gask L, Dowrick C, Towey M, et al. What Do Patients Choose to Tell Their Doctors? Qualitative Analysis of Potential Barriers to Reattributing Medically Unexplained Symptoms. J Gen Intern Med 2008 Dec 17.

[240] Nielsen J, Hansen MS, Fink P. Use of complementary therapy among internal medical inpatients. Prevalence, costs and association with mental disorders and physical diseases. J Psychosom Res 2003 Dec;55(6):547-52.

[241] Waldram J. The efficacy of traditional medicine: Current theoretical and methodological issues. Medical Anthropology Quarterly 2011;14(4):603-25.

[242] Crandon-Malamud L. From the fat of our souls. Social change, political process and medical pluralism in bolivia. University of California Press; 1991.

[243] Brogaard Kristensen D. The shaman or the doctor? Patietn culture and power in southern Chile Copenhagen University; 2008.

[244] Kleinman A. Patients and Healers in the Context of Culture. An Exploration of the Bordeland between Anthropology, Medicine and Psychiatry. University of California Press; 1980.

[245] Kleinman A, Sung. Why do indigenous practitioners successfully heal? Social Science & Medicine 1979;13b:7-26.

[246] Kleinman AM. Writing at the margin: Discourse between anthropology and medicine. University of California Press; 1995.

[247] Mayou R, Bass C, Sharpe M. Treatment of Functional Somatic Symptoms. Oxford, New York, Tokyo: Oxford University Press; 1995.

[248] WHO. The ICD-10 Classification of Mental and Behavioural Disorders. Clinical descriptions and diagnostic guidelines. Geneva: World Health Organization; 1992.

[249] American Psychiatric Association. Diagnostic and Statistical Manual of Mental Disorders (DSM-III). 3 ed. Washington DC: American Psychiatric Association; 1980.

[250] Lipowski ZJ. Somatization: the experience and communication of psychological distress as somatic symptoms. Psychother Psychosom 1987;47:160-7.

[251] Trimble MR. Functional diseases. Br Med J Clin Res Ed 1982 Dec 18;285(6357):1768-70.

[252] Veith I. Hysteria. The History of a Disease. Chicago & London: Phoneix books. The University of Chicago Press; 1965.

[253] Merskey H. The analysis of hysteria. London: Bailliére Tindall; 1979.

[254] Micale MS. Hysteria and its historiography: the future perspective. Hist Psychiatry 1990;33-124.

[255] Fink P. Somatization from a historical perspective. Nord J Psychiatry 1996;50:353-63.

[256] Friendenreich A. Kortfattet speciel Psykiatri. Kjøbenhavn: F.H. Eibes Boghandel; 1901.

[257] Wimmer A. Speciel Klinisk Psykiatri for studerende og læger. København: Levin & Munksgaard.; 1936.

[258] Guze SB, Perley MJ. Observations on The natural history of hysteria. Am J Psychiatry 1963;119:960-5.

[259] Perley MJ, Guze SB. Hysteria- The stability and usefulness of clinical criteria. A Quantitativ Study based on a Follow-up period of six to eight Years in 39 Patients. N Engl J Med 1962;266:421-6.

[260] Fenichel O. The psychoanalytic theory of neurosis. New York, London: W.W.Norton & Company; 1945.

[261] Breuer J, Freud S. Studies on hysteria. The complete psychological Works of Freud. Vol 2. London: Hogarth Press; 1955.

[262] Rodin GM. Somatization: a perspective from self psychology. J Am Acad Psychoanal 1991;19:367-84.

[263] McDougall J. The Psychosoma and the Psychoanalytic process. Int Rev Psycho Anal 1974;1:437-59.

[264] Kohut H. Introspection, empathy, and the semi-circle of mental health. Int J Psychoanal 1982;63:395-407.

[265] Meares R. Stimulus entrapment: On a common basis of somatization. Psychoanalytic Inquiry 1997;17(2):223-34.

[266] Fink P. Physical complaints and symptoms of somatizing patients. J Psychosom Res 1992;36:125-36.

[267] Slater E. Diagnosis of 'hysteria'. BMJ 1965;i:1395-9.

[268] Baglivi G. The Practice of Physic, reduc'd to the ancient Way of Observations, containing a just Parallel between the Wisdom of the Ancients and the Hypothesis's of Modern Physicans. 2nd ed. London (quoted from Veith,I.1965): Midwinter, Linton, Strahan, etc.; 1723.

[269] Lipowski ZJ. Psychosomatic medicine: Past and present. Part I-III. Can J Psychiatry 1986;31:2-13.

[270] Engel GL, Schmale AH. Psychoanalytic therory of somatic disorder. Conversion, specificity and the Disease Onset Situtation. J Am Psychoanal Assoc 1967;15:344-65.

[271] Alexander F. Psychosomatic medicine. Its Principles and Applications. First edition. ed. Mew York: W.W. Norton & Company inc.; 1950.

[272] Thomä H, Kächele H. Psychoanalytic Practice. Berlin, Heidelberg, New York, London, Paris, Tokyo, HongKong, Barcelona, Budapest.: Springer-Verlag; 1992.

[273] Wolff HG. Stress and disease. Springfield: Charles C. Thomas; 1953.

[274] Fink P. Konsultations-liaison psykiatri -psykosomatikkens kliniske pendant. Ugeskr laeger 1994;156(41):6006-10.

[275] Purtell JJ, Robins E, Cohen ME. Observation of Clinical Aspects of Hysteria. A Quantitative Study of 50 Hysteria patients and 156 control subjects. JAMA 1951;146:902-9.

[276] Robins E, O'Neal P. Clinical features of Hysteria in children with a note on prognosis. A two to seventeen year Follow-up study of 41 patients. Nerv Child 1953;10:246-71.

[277] Feighner JP, Robins E, Guze SB, Woodruff Jr RA, Winokur G, Munoz R. Diagnostic criteria for use in psychiatric research. Arch Gen Psychiatry 1972;26:57-63.

[278] Spitzer RL, Endicott J, Robins E. Research diagnostic criteria: rationale and reliability. Arch Gen Psychiatry 1978 Jun;35(6):773-82.

[279] Hansen EB. Paranoia Hypochondriaca. København: Rigshospitalet, Psykiatrisk afd. O; 1976.

[280] Kenyon FE. Hypochondriasis:a survey of some historical, clinical and social aspects. Br J Med Psychol 1965;38:117-33.

[281] Kaplan ML, Asnis GM, Lipschitz DS, Chorney P. Suicidal behavior and abuse in psychiatric outpatients. Compr Psychiatry 1995;36(3):229-35.

[282] Kellner R. Psychosomatic syndromes and somatic symptoms. Washington, London: American Psychiatric Press, Inc.; 1991.

[283] Shorter E. Chronic fatigue in historical perspective. Ciba Found Symp 1993;173:6-16.

[284] Wessely S. Chronic fatigue syndrome: a 20th century illness? Scand J Work Environ Health 1997;23 Suppl 3:17-34:17-34.

[285] Holmes GP, Kaplan JE, Gantz NM, Komaroff AL, Schonberger LB, Straus SE, et al. Chronic fatigue syndrome: a working case definition. Ann Intern Med 1988;108:387-9.

[286] Manu P, Lane TJ, Matthews DA. Chronic fatigue and chronic fatigue syndrome: clinical epidemiology and aetiological classification. Ciba Found Symp 1993;173:23-31.

[287] Sharpe M. Fatigue and chronic fatigue syndrome. Cur Op Psychiat 1992;5(2):207-12.

[288] Wessely S, Sharpe M. Chronic fatigue, chroniuc fatigue syndrome, and fibromyalgia. In: Mayou R, Bass C, Sharpe M, editors. Treatment of functional somatic symptoms. New York: Oxford University Press Inc.; 1995: 285-313.

[289] Wierus J. Joannis Wieri illustrissimi Ducis Julioe Clevioe etc., quondam archiatri, Opera omnia…. (quoted from Veith,I.1965): Apeud Petrum vanden Berge, sub signo Montis Parnassi; 1660.

[290] Carter RB. On the Pathology and Treatment of Hysteria. London: John Churchill; 1853.

[291] Michelsen K. Rachel Hertz' gåde. Kritik,Gyldendal 1984;69:52-86.

[292] Wimmer A. Om Begrebet "Rentehysteri". Tidskrift for arbejdsforsikring 1907;(3.årg.):161-98.

[293] Welner J. Hvad, når man gennemskuer. In: Behrendt P, editor. Kritik.København: Gyldendahl; 1969:89-97.

[294] Falsk læge i fængsel. 39 årig snød flere apoteker i Odense. Ekstra Bladet 1989;10.

[295] American Psychiatric Association. Diagnostic and Statistical Manual of Mental Disorders (DSM-III-R). Washington, DC.: APA; 1987.

[296] Asher R. Munchausen's syndrome. Lancet 1951;1:339-41.

[297] Patterson R. The Münchausen syndrome: Baron von Münchausen has taken a bum rap. CMAJ 1988;139(Sep.15):566-9.

[298] Sternbach RA. Varieties of Pain Games. Adv Neurol 1974;4:423-430.

Supplementary material

Patient materials

Fjorback LO. Mindfulness. PsykiatriFonden; 2011. (Patient guide with cd). An English translation can be acquired from The Research Clinic for Functional Disorders on request.

Leaflets

Bodily Distress Syndrome. Information about BDS for patients and relatives. The Research Clinic for Functional Disorders, 2012.

Homepages

www.functionaldisorders.dk (information and materials for both professionals, patients and relatives.

Supplementary reading

Creed F, Henningsen P, Fink P (Eds). Medically unexplained symptoms, somatisation and bodily distress. Developing better clinical services. Cambridge University Press; 2011.

Fink P. Somatization disorder and related disorders. In: Gelder MG, Andreasen N, Lopez-Ibor JJ, Geddes JR, editors. New Oxford Textbook of Psychiatry. 2nd ed. Oxford University Press Inc., New York; 2009. p. 999-1011.

Woolfolk RL, Allen LA. Treating somatization. A cognitive-behavioral approach. New York: The Guilford Press; 2007.

Appendices

Appendix 1
Weekly registration form

For each day and each time of the day, please indicate the severity of your symptoms on the below scale:

No pain/
discomfort/   0 1 2 3 4 5 6 7 8 9 10   Worst possible
emotions   pain/discomfort/
                                                               emotions

For each entry, please write one or two words about the situation you were in when you had the symptoms. This could, for instance, be "on the bus", "at work", "while visiting my mother in law", etc.

	day date:	day date:	day date:	day date:	day date:	day date:	day date:
Morning							
Afternoon							
Late afternoon							
Night							

Appendix 2
CMDQ Index (Common Mental Disorders Questionnaire)

During the last 4 weeks how much were you bothered by:	Not at all	A little	Moderately	Quite a bit	Extremely
1. Headaches?	0	1	2	3	4
2. Dizziness or faintness?	0	1	2	3	4
3. Pains in heart or cheast?	0	1	2	3	4
4. Pains in lower back?	0	1	2	3	4
5. Nausea or upset stomach?	0	1	2	3	4
6. Soreness of your muscles?	0	1	2	3	4
7. Trouble getting your breath?	0	1	2	3	4
8. Hot or cold spells?	0	1	2	3	4
9. Numbness or tingling in parts of your body?	0	1	2	3	4
10. A lump in your throat?	0	1	2	3	4
11. Feeling weak in parts of your body?	0	1	2	3	4
12. Heavy feelings in your arms or legs?	0	1	2	3	4
13. Worries that there is something seriously wrong with your body?	0	1	2	3	4
14. Worries that you suffer a disease you have read or heard about?	0	1	2	3	4
15. Many different pains and aches?	0	1	2	3	4
16. Worries about the possibility of having a serious illness?	0	1	2	3	4
17. Many different symptoms?	0	1	2	3	4

18. Thoughts that the doctor may be wrong if telling you not to worry?	0	1	2	3	4
19. Worries about your health?	0	1	2	3	4
20. Feeling suddenly scared for no reason?	0	1	2	3	4
21. Nervousness or shaki-ness inside?	0	1	2	3	4
22. Spells of terror or panic?	0	1	2	3	4
23. You worry too much?	0	1	2	3	4
24. Feeling blue?	0	1	2	3	4
25. Feelings of worthless-ness?	0	1	2	3	4
26. Thoughts of ending your life?	0	1	2	3	4
27. Feelings of being trapped or caught?	0	1	2	3	4
28. Feeling lonely?	0	1	2	3	4
29. Blaming yourself for things?	0	1	2	3	4

Within the last year, have you ever ...	No	Yes
30. Felt you ought to cut down on your drinking?	0	1
31. Been annoyed by people criticizing your drinking?	0	1
32. Felt bad or guilty about your drinking?	0	1
33. Had a drink in the morning to steady your nerves or get rid of a hangover?	0	1

Normal values CMDQ:
Symptom check list (item 1-12): <6
Health anxiety (item 13-19): <2
Anxiety disorder (item 20-23): <2
Depressive disorder (item 24-29): <3
Alkohol problem (item 30-33): <2

Appendix 3
Problem-solving model

1) What is your problem?

2) What will you have achieved once you have solved our problem?

3) Describe *various* ways in which this problem may be solved (use your imagination).

4) For each way in which the problem may be solved, consider the pros and cons. Finally, choose the best or more realistic solution to your problem.

5) The way you have decided to solve your problem should be divided into steps or partial objectives/tasks (see Steps of objectives) Make sure these are realistic and that you are capable of taking each individual step. Describe how you will take each step and when you aim to have achieved your objective.

6) You will make an agreement with yourself or with some other person on how and when you will take each individual step.

7) What could stop you from taking the steps you have planned? What can you do to ensure that you are successful?

8) Next time, consider if you took the planned steps and if the next steps need to be adjusted.

Appendix 4 A-B
Automatic and alternative thoughts ad behaviour model

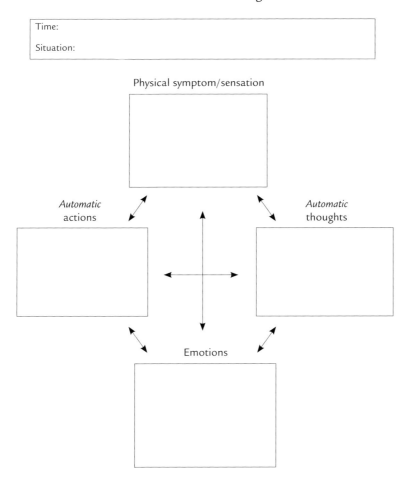

Basic model 1 with *automatic* thoughts and actions

Time:

Situation:

Physical symptom/sensation

Automatic
actions

Automatic
thoughts

Emotions

Basic model 2 with *alternative* thoughts or actions

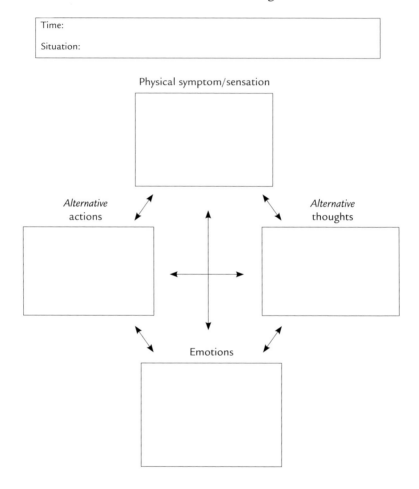

Time:

Situation:

Physical symptom/sensation

Alternative actions

Alternative thoughts

Emotions

Appendix 5
Illness and symptom interpretation

Possible causes of your illness and symptoms:

Causes (1)	What supports your explanation (symptoms?)	What contradicts your explanation?	What are the consequences if you are right? (2)*

(1) Rank causes by adding "1" by the most important cause, "2" by the second most important cause, etc.
(2) What are the implications of this for your thoughts, behaviour and treatment if this is the right cause? What can you do yourself? How will you manage this situation?
* If more relevant, this issue may be addressed through the question: "How can you find out what the consequences are?"

Appendix 6
Steps of objectives

Introduction: Please fill in below.
1. Fill in the objective of your treatment participation at the uppermost step.
2. At the various steps, add the partial objectives on your way to the final objective.
   Note! Objectives should be realistic!

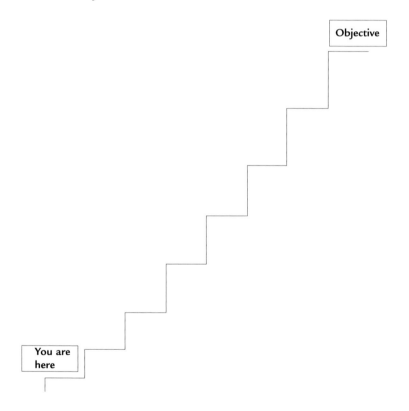

Appendix 7
List of objectives

For each group of objectives (i.e. physical objectives, social objectives, work-life objectives, other objectives) state at least one objectives you want to reach.

In order to reach these objectives, they must be realistic and concrete. For example an exercise objective could be:
1. "To go for a walk for 15 minutes every morning from 10AM to 10.15AM"
2. "To do a relaxation exercise for 10 minutes every morning from 9AM to 9.10AM"

A. Physical objectives
1. Exercise _____ _____
   _____
   _____
   _____

2. Increase muscles _____
   _____
   _____
   _____

3. Relaxation exercise _____
   _____
   _____
   _____

B. Social/leisure objectives
1. Socialt _____
   _____
   _____
   _____

2. Family _____
   _____
   _____
   _____

3. Leisure time _____
   _____
   _____
   _____

C. Work-life/occupational objectives
1. _____
   _____
   _____
   _____

2. _____
   _____
   _____
   _____

3. _____
   _____
   _____
   _____

D. Other objectives
1. _____
   _____
   _____
   _____

2. _____
   _____
   _____
   _____

3. _____
   _____
   _____
   _____

Appendix 8
Two-stage pathway model – children

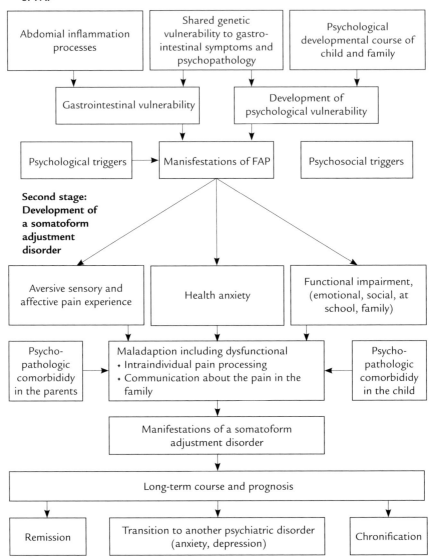

First stage development of FAP

Abdomial inflammation processes	Shared genetic vulnerability to gastro-intestinal symptoms and psychopathology	Psychological developmental course of child and family

Gastrointestinal vulnerability

Development of psychological vulnerability

Psychological triggers → Manisfestations of FAP

Psychosocial triggers

Second stage: Development of a somatoform adjustment disorder

Aversive sensory and affective pain experience

Health anxiety

Functional impairment, (emotional, social, at school, family)

Psycho-pathologic comorbididy in the parents →

Maladaption including dysfunctional
+ Intraindividual pain processing
+ Communication about the pain in the family

← Psycho-pathologic comorbididy in the child

Manifestations of a somatoform adjustment disorder

Long-term course and prognosis

Remission

Transition to another psychiatric disorder (anxiety, depression)

Chronification

Appendix 9
CSI – parents report

Your child's symptoms

The list below features symptoms often seen in children and teenagers. Please consider each symptom and tick off the number that shows how much your child has been bothered by each of these symptoms over the past 2 weeks.

How much has your child been bothered by each of the below symptoms over the past 2 weeks?

	Not at all	A little	Some what	Much	Very much
1. Headache	0	1	2	3	4
2. Faintness or dizziness (feeling faint or dizzy)	0	1	2	3	4
3. Pain in heart or chest	0	1	2	3	4
4. Feeling of being without energy or being slower	0	1	2	3	4
5. Pain in lower part of back	0	1	2	3	4
6. Sore muscles	0	1	2	3	4
7. Difficulty in breathing (other than when the child is doing exercise)	0	1	2	3	4
8. Sweats or chills (suddenly feeling warm or cold for no reason)	0	1	2	3	4
9. Numbness or tingling in parts of the body	0	1	2	3	4
10. A lump in the throat	0	1	2	3	4
11. Weakness (to feel weak) in parts of the body	0	1	2	3	4
12. Feeling of a bearing down sensation in arms or legs (feel too heavy to move)	0	1	2	3	4
13. Nausea or feeling of uneasiness in stomach	0	1	2	3	4

	Not at all	A little	Some what	Much	Very much
14. Constipation (when it is difficult to pass stools)	0	1	2	3	4
15. Loose stools or diarrhoea	0	1	2	3	4
16. Abdominal or pelvic pain (stomach ache)	0	1	2	3	4
17. Heart beats too fast (even when the child is not doing exercise)	0	1	2	3	4
18. Difficulty swallowing	0	1	2	3	4
19. Lost voice	0	1	2	3	4
20. Deafness (when child cannot hear)	0	1	2	3	4
21. Double vision (when child sees two of everything while wearing glasses)	0	1	2	3	4
22. Blurred vision (when things are blurred even when child wears glasses)	0	1	2	3	4
23. Blindness (the child cannot see)	0	1	2	3	4
24. Fainting	0	1	2	3	4
25. Loss of memory or amnesia (lost memory, cannot remember things)	0	1	2	3	4
26. Seizures or cramps (body moves or shakes, cannot control movements)	0	1	2	3	4
27. Difficulty walking	0	1	2	3	4
28. Paralysis or muscular fatigue (muscles too weak to move)	0	1	2	3	4
29. Difficulty urinating (peeing)	0	1	2	3	4
30. Vomiting	0	1	2	3	4
31. Feeling bloated	0	1	2	3	4
32. Food makes your child sick	0	1	2	3	4

	Not at all	A little	Some what	Much	Very much
33. Pain in knees, elbows other joints	0	1	2	3	4
34. Pain in arms and legs	0	1	2	3	4
35. Pain upon urinating or peeing	0	1	2	3	4
36. Only girls. Has your daughter had her period within the past two weeks?		YES		NO	
37. Only girls. If yes, where the symptoms she told about related to her period?	0	1	2	3	4

* A standardised measure for Danish children has not been published. The below table lists parent-reported SCI scores (average, median and standard deviation (SD)) for American populations of children referred to specialist treatment for diagnostic assessment of suspected recurrent functional abdominal pain) and healthy children, respectively (age range 6-18 years; largely equal gender distribution, girls mainly Caucasian). On the basis of these figures, we may cautiously argue that a score > 20 supports a diagnosis of functional symptoms. However, it should be noted that the total score may vary according to age and gender.

Population	N	Average	Median	SD	Range
Clinical population	493	20.04	17.00	12.37	0-90
Healthy population	54	5.73	3.00	7.41	0-37

Index